Field Guide to

the Business of Medicine

Resource for Health Care Professionals

Field Guide to
the Business of Medicine
Resource for Health Care Professionals

Christopher A. Clyne, MD, MBA
Diplomate of the American Board of Internal Medicine
Fellow of the American Heart Association
Fellow of the American College of Cardiology
Fellow of the Heart Rhythm Society
Barrington, Rhode Island

Britton Jewell, DO, MHA
Fellow in the American College of Osteopathic Internists
Rockville, Maryland

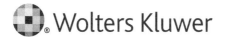 Wolters Kluwer

Philadelphia • Baltimore • New York • London
Buenos Aires • Hong Kong • Sydney • Tokyo

Acquisitions Editor: Rebecca Gaertner
Manager, Books Editorial Coordinators: Annette Ferran
Marketing Manager: Rachel Mante-Leung
Production Project Manager: Bridgett Dougherty
Design Coordinator: Holly McLaughlin
Manufacturing Coordinator: Beth Welsh
Prepress Vendor: S4Carlisle Publishing Services

9 8 7 6 5 4 3 2 1

Printed in China

Library of Congress Cataloging-in-Publication Data

Names: Clyne, Christopher A., editor. | Jewell, Britton, editor.
Title: Field guide to the business of medicine: resource for health care
    professionals / edited by Christopher A. Clyne, Britton Jewell.
Description: First edition. | Philadelphia, PA: Wolters Kluwer, 2019. |
    Includes index.
Identifiers: LCCN 2018031932 | ISBN 9781496396235 (pbk.)
Subjects: | MESH: Practice Management, Medical
Classification: LCC R728 | NLM W 80 | DDC 610.68—dc23
    LC record available at https://lccn.loc.gov/2018031932

shop.lww.com

Dedication

This book is for all who have dedicated their lives to taking care of those in need. Their commitment to meeting the health care challenges of a changing world makes us proud to be called colleagues.

Christopher A. Clyne and Britton Jewell

Contributors

Mark D. Carlson, MD, MA
Adjunct Professor of Medicine
Department of Medicine
Case Western Reserve University
Cleveland, Ohio
Chief Medical Officer and Division Vice President
Cardiovascular and Neuromodulation
Abbott
Sylmar, California

Christopher A. Clyne, MD, MBA
Diplomate of the American Board of Internal Medicine
Fellow of the American Heart Association
Fellow of the American College of Cardiology
Fellow of the Heart Rhythm Society
Barrington, Rhode Island

Britton Jewell, DO, MHA
Fellow in the American College of Osteopathic Internists
Rockville, Maryland

Carla Martin, MD
Internal/Medicine Pediatrics Physician
Providence Community Health Centers
Clinical Assistant Professor of Family Medicine
Brown University School of Medicine
Providence, Rhode Island

Foreword

In the late 20th century, Sister Irene Kraus, a nun who became the founding Chief Executive of the Daughters of Charity National Health System, was credited for coining the phrase "no Margin, no Mission." Over the past three decades, not-for-profit medical institutions have slowly and begrudgingly accepted that fact that in order to fulfill their mission (or even to continue to exist for that matter), they have no choice but to be fiscally responsible. Concerns about profitability are no longer only designated to hospital administrators but are more and more a prerequisite in hiring successful physician leaders, including deans, hospital department chiefs, and even research directors. The days of academic chairs being selected solely on the strengths of their publication lists and successes in obtaining grants are now long past. Furthermore, many hospital CEOs are now business-trained physicians who often have obtained MBAs.

Yet, as these changes have occurred "at the top," medical school and residency education has woefully lagged in preparing future doctors in even the basic fundamentals of the business of health care. The primer *Field Guide to the Business of Medicine: Resource for Health Care Professionals* has been long overdue and should be required reading for all physicians in training.

Deeb N. Salem, MD
Physician-in-Chief
Tufts Medical Center

Preface

A few years ago, a colleague opined that medicine in the 1980s was "fun," but that today's medicine was so laden with forms, deadlines, and contracts that he had no time to enjoy the practice of medicine. I realized then that many were unprepared for all of the business-related requirements for today's practitioners.

Around the same time, I met a young doctor who was keenly interested in the business side of medicine. We realized that there was a need to educate practitioners and administrators in some of the important aspects of health care not covered in school curricula or training programs. We hope that this book serves as a valued resource for those soon to be, or currently are, in the delivery of health care in the United States.

Christopher A. Clyne, MD, MBA

Acknowledgments

Special thanks to our families, without whose support and patience this work would not have been possible, and to the editorial team at Wolters Kluwer, who kept us on point and were valued partners.

Christopher A. Clyne, MD, MBA
Britton Jewell, DO, MHA

Contents

Business of Health Care 101
Introduction

Christopher A. Clyne, MD, MBA
Britton Jewell, DO, MHA

Congratulations! You were at the top of your high school and college graduation classes. You aced Organic and "killed" the Medical College Admission Test (MCAT), Dental Admission Test (DAT), or Graduate Record Examinations (GRE). You got into medical/dental/graduate school and finished your training. Now you have to decide how to "practice" in the medical universe. Well, here is where things get really complicated.

You are well prepared to diagnose and cure disease and plan for success, but did you plan on spending hours on credentialing or planning your schedule and/or budgeting for the new electronic health record (EHR) system your office or hospital will purchase? How will this impact your patient load, productivity, and free time? What are the quality metrics for your specialty or organization? Should you join a private group or be employed? How are you to be paid? Is your organization solid? Are your benefits competitive? What is an accountable care organization (ACO)? What does the Affordable Care Act (ACA) actually do?

These are important questions that are not part of the (pre)medical/professional school curriculum or medical training for most practitioners and allied health professionals. We combined our experiences as a new graduate looking forward and an experienced physician learning new systems, to construct this *Field Guide to the Business of Medicine* as a resource for health care professionals. We provide a composite of many of the business and administrative challenges that you may not have faced in school and training but that will be a significant consumer of time and energy in the practice of medicine now and for the future. This field guide will be a valuable resource for the uninitiated, unprepared, and un-savvy health care professional.

Fundamentals of Health Insurance
Medicare and Medicaid

Christopher A. Clyne, MD, MBA
Britton Jewell, DO, MHA

Medicare and Medicaid are government-run insurance plans. It is impossible to make it through your health care training without encountering these programs, and they will have a huge impact on you throughout your career. In fact, there is no other entity that shapes the U.S. health care economy as much as these programs do. Keeping that in mind, this chapter will focus on the major differences between these programs and will discuss how they reimburse hospitals and providers.

WHAT ARE THE DIFFERENCES BETWEEN MEDICARE AND MEDICAID?

In general, Medicare is under federal control, whereas Medicaid has both federal and state government oversight. Medicare typically provides services for older Americans, and Medicaid provides services for those individuals under 65 years with incomes up to 133% of the federal poverty level.

Medicare

Medicare is government-sponsored health insurance for select groups of individuals (Figure 1-1):

- Those 65 years of age or older
- Those under 65 years with select disabilities (have to receive Social Security Disability benefits for at least 2 years)

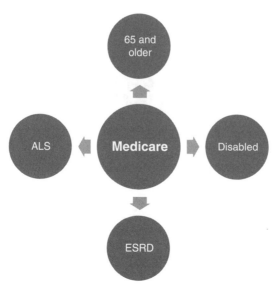

Figure 1-1 Groups of individuals eligible for Medicare. ALS, amyotrophic lateral sclerosis; ESRD, end-stage renal disease.

■ Those with end-stage renal disease or amyotrophic lateral sclerosis regardless of age

Medicare is divided up into four parts termed A, B, C, and D (Figure 1-2).

Medicare Part A principally provides not only hospital insurance but also coverage for inpatient skilled nursing facilities (SNFs), inpatient psychiatric care, home health care, and hospice services. Medicare Part A is premium free for eligible individuals as long as they or their spouse paid Medicare taxes (which is almost everyone), but are still subject to deductibles. In 2018, the annual deductible was $1,340.

Medicare Part B provides medical insurance for outpatient doctor's visits, preventative care, other outpatient tests, home health care, outpatient psychiatric care, and durable medical equipment (DME). Patients who are admitted to hospital as "Observation" status under Medicare B will be responsible for a 20% deductible. Private supplement insurance policies may be purchased to cover this

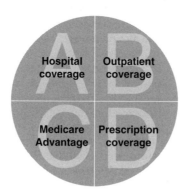

Figure 1-2 The components of Medicare.

20%. Medicare Part B requires a standard monthly premium, deductible, and 20% coinsurance. In 2018, the annual deductible was $183 and the standard monthly premium was $134. Preventative care services including a yearly checkup are included with no additional charge.

Medicare Part C is also called Medicare Advantage. This program allows private insurance companies to provide Medicare Part A, Part B, and usually Part D benefits all in one package through different plan options such as a preferred provider organization (PPO) or a health maintenance organization (HMO) insurance plan. These plans typically provide better value and include more benefits than the standard plan with little or no additional premium cost. These private insurers are paid by Medicare to provide services to enrollees. In 2015, over one-third of Medicare enrollees were covered under this type of plan.

Medicare Part D provides prescription drug benefits supplied by private insurance companies. These plans are subject to premiums, deductibles, and coinsurance that vary for each plan.

Doctor's and other practitioner's services are covered by Medicare Part A or B, depending on the setting. Medicare not only reimburses the majority of physicians through a fee-for-service model, but may also pay hospitals, SNFs, home health companies, hospice facilities, and many other health care providers directly. In addition, Medicare pays private health plans that provide Part C and Part D benefits. Medicare reimbursement schemes for both hospitals and providers are discussed in more detail in subsequent chapters.

Medigap

You may have heard the term *Medigap*, which refers to Medicare Supplement Insurance provided by private insurance companies. This type of insurance has a separate monthly premium that helps to cover the "gaps" in Medicare, as the standard coverage is far from comprehensive. These plans help cover deductibles, copayments, and coinsurance. For example, Medigap may cover the extra 20% coinsurance typically paid out of pocket by enrollees. To be eligible for Medigap, enrollees must have Original Medicare coverage and not be covered under a Medicare Advantage plan.

Medicaid

Medicaid provides insurance coverage for those who cannot afford it (Figure 1-3). As stated earlier, both federal and state governments are involved with financing this program. Medicaid also provides additional coverage for long-term care services that are not covered by Medicare.

Medicaid eligibility requires low income in addition to one of the following categories:

- Adults 65 years of age and older
- Children under 19 years
- Pregnant women
- Disabled individuals

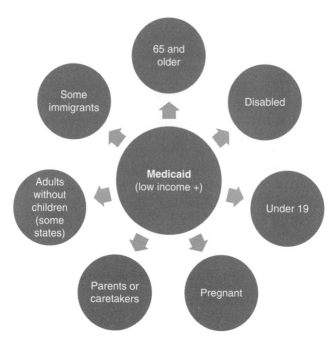

Figure 1-3 Groups of individuals eligible for Medicaid.

- Parents or adults caring for children
- Adults without children (mostly in states that expanded Medicaid coverage under the Affordable Care Act)
- Some immigrants

Medicaid provides similar benefits to Medicare Part A, Part B, and Part D. It provides coverage for inpatient hospital services, outpatient physician services, long-term care, preventative care services, and medications. Of note, neither Medicaid nor Medicare offers dental or vision services for adults. Medicaid does provide dental and vision coverage for children.

Dual Eligible Beneficiaries

The group of individuals who are eligible for both Medicare and Medicaid are termed dual eligible. For these enrollees, Medicaid provides assistance with paying the premiums, coinsurance, and copayments for Medicare benefits. Therefore, Medicaid acts as a form of supplemental insurance in these cases. In 2010, there were 10 million individuals covered under both plans. This group is very expensive to cover because they accounted for over one-third of spending each for Medicare and Medicaid but only made up 20% of Medicare and 14% of Medicaid enrollees in 2010. Because of their excessive cost, they have been the subject of increased focus to reduce health care spending.

HOW DOES MEDICARE PAY HOSPITALS?

The Centers for Medicare & Medicaid Services (CMS) has established a Prospective Payment System (PPS) that is used to reimburse hospitals, SNFs, home health companies, hospices, outpatient hospital services, inpatient rehabilitation, inpatient psychiatric facilities, and long-term care hospitals. The prospective system was put into place because of the skyrocketing costs under the previous retrospective system, which reimbursed for services that were already provided. Because of this, CMS has established a predetermined amount to reimburse depending on the classification of the care provided, which helps control costs. Acute inpatient hospital services are reimbursed according to the inpatient PPS (IPPS) that uses diagnosis-related groups (DRGs) and outpatient hospital services are reimbursed according to the outpatient PPS (OPPS) that uses ambulatory payment classifications (APCs).

Inpatient Prospective Payment System and Diagnosis-Related Groups

The IPPS uses DRGs to combine similar medical conditions and their associated procedures during a hospitalization, which can be altered by the patient's age, gender, comorbidities, or discharge disposition. The DRGs are assigned at discharge so that analogous cases can be expected to require the same level of care and therefore receive the same reimbursement. The final DRG is composed of the primary diagnosis and up to 24 secondary diagnoses, termed complications or comorbidities. The current reimbursement system is called the Medicare Severity-DRG, which provides for three different levels of severity to determine the secondary diagnoses. A secondary diagnosis can be classified as a Major Complication or Comorbidity (MCC) that raises the DRG reimbursement the most, followed by a Complication or Comorbidity (CC), and then a non–Complication or Comorbidity (non-CC), which does not alter reimbursement as much. It is for this reason that most hospitals have a clinical documentation improvement (CDI) department that reviews charts and sends you frequent queries in order to clarify or add to your documentation to maximize the DRG for billing purposes. See Chapter 4 for further information on how the DRG system affects hospital reimbursement.

Adjustments to Inpatient Reimbursement

CMS is moving away from a fee-for-service model, where providers are reimbursed for each episode of care, and is moving toward a model that incentivizes quality. CMS has established several programs to accomplish this. They are listed briefly here and are discussed in greater detail in Chapter 4.

The major programs that affect a hospital's reimbursement are as follows:

- Hospital Value-Based Purchasing (VBP) Program
- Hospital Readmissions Reduction Program
- Hospital-Acquired Condition (HAC) Reduction Program

The Hospital VBP Program is funded by a 2% reduction of all DRG reimbursements, which are then paid back to the hospitals on the basis of performance in certain quality areas, such as patient safety. The Hospital Readmissions Reduction Program can reduce overall payments of up to 3% for hospitals that perform poorly with reportable readmissions for diagnoses such as heart failure. The Hospital Acquired Condition (HAC) Reduction Program can reduce overall payments by 1% for hospitals that are in the bottom 25% for HACs, such as catheter-associated urinary tract infections.

Therefore, avoiding these penalties is very important for the institution's future financial solvency. Understanding these clinical quality benchmarks serves to help focus attention on providing the necessary excellent patient care and proper documentation.

The hospital's reimbursement will also be increased if it is a teaching hospital, cares for a disproportionate share of poor patients, uses certain new technology, or has very expensive outlier cases.

Outpatient Prospective Payment System and Ambulatory Payment Classifications

The OPPS uses APCs in a similar manner as DRGs. As the name suggests, this system is used by Medicare to reimburse for hospital outpatient services, and it can also be used to make payments for some Part B inpatient services not covered by Part A, partial hospitalization services, some Durable Medical Equipment (DME), and some drugs. The APC combines the major components of a service into the payment, which may include, but are not restricted to, ancillary services, supplies, laboratory work, anesthesia, operating room costs, implantable devices, and some drugs. Some procedures are completely included in an APC, such as an incision and drainage. To reimburse for services, CMS attributes the Healthcare Common Procedure Coding System (HCPCS) codes (discussed later) to an APC to determine the amount. Reimbursements can be adjusted on the basis of several factors including the reporting of quality measures and the hospital location.

Healthcare Common Procedure Coding System

To understand Medicare reimbursement schemes, it is important to have a working knowledge of the HCPCS. The HCPCS is the system of billing codes used by Medicare and other private insurance companies and is divided into two sets, namely, Level I and Level II. Level I is made up of the Current Procedural Terminology (CPT) coding system, which is owned and managed by the American Medical Association (AMA). This is very powerful—it is why the AMA is a vital part of the CMS payment system. Because they own the coding system, they are a necessary player in establishing physician payment. This system is used by physicians and other health care providers to bill for procedures and services. Level II is the system used to bill for everything else, such as supplies, drugs, and DME, and is managed by CMS.

If you are employed by a hospital or have privileges at a hospital, they will care most about accurate documentation and preventing readmissions and HACs.

Therefore, make sure you are documenting how sick the patient is in real life on paper with accurate diagnoses so the CDI specialists can code for the most accurate (and highest) DRG or APC. Also, make sure you document if the condition was "present on admission" to avoid any ambiguity regarding HACs. A lot of physicians today are salaried employees, and so their income is not affected by the factors mentioned earlier. Nevertheless, you should want to keep your employer happy! Understanding this section will allow you to do that.

HOW DOES MEDICARE PAY PROVIDERS?

CMS has established a Medicare Physician Fee Schedule that governs how physicians and other health care providers are paid under Medicare Part B. Both inpatient and outpatient providers are paid in this fee-for-service manner.

Medicare Physician Fee Schedule

In order to receive reimbursement:

- Providers must document the appropriate medical diagnoses using the *International Classification of Diseases* 10th edition–Clinical Modification codes. This is a list of over 144,000 diagnostic descriptions that use specific locations and circumstances to define the reason for the encounter.
- The provider must bill for the appropriate CPT code (see HCPCS section earlier). Procedures have a CPT code already assigned to them, and patient encounter CPT codes are chosen by the provider on the basis of the level of complexity and/or time spent with the patient defined by the Evaluation and Management documentation guidelines established by the CMS.
- CMS then uses the CPT code of each procedure or visit and assigns what is called a relative value unit (RVU) to it on the basis of the amount of resources used in the form of physician work (wRVU), practice expense, and malpractice insurance cost. The RVU varies by physician/surgeon specialty and is further adjusted by what are termed Geographic Practice Cost Indices on the basis of cost differences for varying locations and then multiplied by a conversion factor to come up with the final reimbursement rate. Therefore, CMS sets a standard number of RVUs for each CPT code and for the Medicare reimbursement of each type of patient encounter and procedure.

CMS is responsible for managing and updating the RVUs. This is done on a regular basis in conjunction with the AMA, which owns the CPT codes. RVUs are important for physicians to understand because some employed physicians receive bonuses or are paid partially by the amount of wRVUs they generate. Figure 1-4 provides a representation of how the initial patient encounter becomes the final payment.

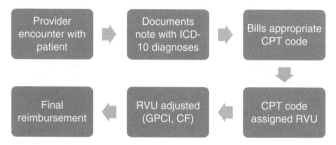

Figure 1-4 How Medicare pays providers. CF, conversion factor; CPT, current procedural terminology; GPCI, geographic practice cost indices; *ICD-10, International Classification of Diseases* 10th edition; RVU, relative value unit. Adapted from the Medicare Access and CHIP Reauthorization Act of 2015.

The Medicare Access and CHIP Reauthorization Act of 2015

The Sustainable Growth Rate was a system of payment created by the CMS in 1997 as an attempt to control Medicare spending by limiting payment to physicians. The goal of this legislation was to keep Medicare spending neutral by reducing (or increasing) physician payment for Medicare patients on the basis of the previous year's gross domestic product. This calculus resulted in predicted cuts to doctors most years, with threatened cuts of up to 27.4% (in 2013). From 2003 to 2017, Congress was forced to suspend these cuts 17 times.

As a response, the Medicare Access and CHIP Reauthorization Act of 2015 (MACRA) was passed with bipartisan support and promised to fundamentally change the way the United States evaluates and pays for health care using performance, value, and shared risk as components of the reimbursement equation for providers.

MACRA uses two new performance-based provisions to determine CMS payment (up or down) to doctors and providers (Figure 1-5):

- The Merit-Based Incentive Payment System (MIPS) ties CMS payments to performance on the basis of four dimensions: clinical quality, resource use, health information technology (IT) meaningful use, and clinical practice improvement activities. MIPS consolidates and replaces the Physician Quality Reporting System, the Medicare electronic health record (EHR) Incentive Program (Meaningful Use), and the Value-Based Modifier Program that used to affect physician reimbursement.
- The Alternative Payment Model (APM) is designed to substitute value-based payment for the former "fee-for-service" payment model. Providers may earn up to a 5% incentive bonus from 2019 to 2024, with more aggressive incentives thereafter if they meet criteria on the basis of the patient volume served, use of a certified EHR, employment of established quality measures, and willingness to bear "more than nominal risk" (the cost to restructure). Participants in the APMs would typically

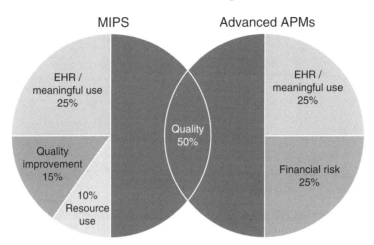

Figure 1-5 The Medicare Access and CHIP Reauthorization Act (MACRA) 2019 weights. APM, alternative payment model; EHR, electronic health record; MIPS, merit-based incentive payment system.

include Accountable Care Organizations, patient-centered medical homes, patient-centered specialty practices, and those providers that employ the episode/bundle-based payment model.

HOW DOES MEDICAID PAY HOSPITALS AND PROVIDERS?

The Medicaid system of reimbursement is not as complex as Medicare. However, the payments are lower. As noted earlier, Medicaid is under both federal and state control. The federal government helps the states pay for some of their Medicaid costs on the basis of the Federal Medical Assistance Percentage that is set for each state. The base rate for Medicaid reimbursements is set by the states and is paid to hospitals and providers in a fee-for-service manner or through managed care. The base rate is not the final payment, however. There is also a complicated system of supplemental payments including items like waivers and taxes. In addition, states send Disproportionate Share Hospital payments to the hospitals that provide care to large amounts of low-income individuals or Medicaid enrollees. The final combination and amount of payments vary from state to state. The relationship between the federal government, the states, and the citizens of each state is under review by the current administration. The payment structure is evolving and may be revised such that states may receive block grants from the Treasury on the basis of the number of Medicaid recipients that qualify in accord with each individual state's eligibility criteria. Distribution of the federal monies would be up to each state.

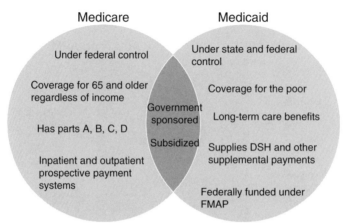

Figure 1-6 Similarities and differences between Medicare and Medicaid. DSH, Disproportionate Share Hospital; FMAP, Federal Medical Assistance Percentage.

CONCLUSION

The health care professional must understand the intersections among all stakeholders (employers, hospitals, providers, patients, the government, industry, and insurance companies) to have a successful enterprise. Whether you are salaried or self-employed, you will achieve a greater appreciation of the value you bring to your corporation when you are familiar with the systems and protocols in place that control the flow of resources in health care. Having a basic understanding of two of the most influential payers in the U.S. health care system is a large part of this. You will also comprehend your administrators better as you are aware of their points of view from a financial perspective. Figure 1-6 summarizes the main parts of this chapter with a comparison of the similarities and differences between Medicare and Medicaid.

Recommended Resources

Blue Cross Blue Shield of Michigan. What Do Medicare Supplement Plans Cover? http://www.bcbsm.com/medicare/help/faqs/works/supplement-plans-cover.html. Updated November 14, 2016. Accessed April 18, 2018.

Centers for Medicare & Medicaid Services. Acute Care Hospital Inpatient Prospective Payment System. CMS.gov. https://www.cms.gov/Outreach-and-Education/Medicare-Learning-Network-MLN/MLNProducts/Downloads/AcutePaymtSysfctsht.pdf. Published December 2016. Accessed April 18, 2018.

Centers for Medicare & Medicaid Services. Evaluation and Management Services. CMS.gov. https://www.cms.gov/Outreach-and-Education/Medicare-Learning-Network-MLN/MLNProducts/Downloads/eval-mgmt-serv-guide-ICN006764.pdf. Published August 2017. Accessed April 18, 2018.

Centers for Medicare & Medicaid Services. Financing. Medicaid.gov. https://www.medicaid.gov/chip/financing/index.html. Accessed April 18, 2018.

Centers for Medicare & Medicaid Services. HCPCS—General Information. CMS.gov. https://www.cms.gov/Medicare/Coding/MedHCPCSGenInfo/index.html. Updated March 23, 2018. Accessed April 18, 2018.

Centers for Medicare & Medicaid Services. Hospital Outpatient Prospective Payment System. CMS.gov. https://www.cms.gov/Outreach-and-Education/Medicare-Learning-Network-MLN/MLNProducts/downloads/HospitalOutpaysysfctsht.pdf. Published December 2017. Accessed April 18, 2018.

Centers for Medicare & Medicaid Services. Hospital Value-Based Purchasing. Medicare.gov. https://www.medicare.gov/hospitalcompare/Data/hospital-vbp.html. Accessed April 18, 2018.

Centers for Medicare & Medicaid Services. Hospital VBP Program Aggregate Payment Adjustments. Medicare.gov. https://www.medicare.gov/HospitalCompare/Data/payment-adjustments.html. Accessed April 18, 2018.

Centers for Medicare & Medicaid Services. Innovation Models. The CMS Innovation Center. https://innovation.cms.gov/initiatives#views=models. Accessed April 18, 2018.

Centers for Medicare & Medicaid Services. Medicare 2018 Costs at a Glance. Medicare.gov. https://www.medicare.gov/your-medicare-costs/costs-at-a-glance/costs-at-a-glance.html. Accessed April 18, 2018.

Centers for Medicare & Medicaid Services. Medicare Physician Fee Schedule. CMS.gov. https://www.cms.gov/Outreach-and-Education/Medicare-Learning-Network-MLN/MLNProducts/downloads/MedcrephysFeeSchedfctsht.pdf. Published February 2017. Accessed April 18, 2018.

Centers for Medicare & Medicaid Services. MIPS Overview. Quality Payment Program. https://qpp.cms.gov/learn/qpp. Accessed April 18, 2018.

Centers for Medicare & Medicaid Services. The Merit-Based Incentive Payment System: MIPS Scoring Methodology Overview. CMS.gov. https://www.cms.gov/Medicare/Quality-Initiatives-Patient-Assessment-Instruments/Value-Based-Programs/MACRA-MIPS-and-APMs/MIPS-Scoring-Methodology-slide-deck.pdf. Accessed April 18, 2018.

Centers for Medicare & Medicaid Services. What's Medicare and Medicaid? Medicare.gov. https://www.medicare.gov/Pubs/pdf/11306-Medicare-Medicaid.pdf. Updated September 2017. Accessed April 18, 2018.

Cubanski J, Swoope C, Boccuti C, et al. A Primer on Medicare: Key Facts About the Medicare Program and the People It Covers. Kaiser Family Foundation. http://files.kff.org/attachment/report-a-primer-on-medicare-key-facts-about-the-medicare-program-and-the-people-it-covers. Published March 2015. Accessed April 18, 2018.

Hawaii State Health Insurance Assistance Program. Frequently Asked Questions. http://www.hawaiiship.org/Portals/_AgencySite/pdf/FAQs.pdf. Accessed April 18, 2018.

Kaiser Family Foundation. An Overview of Medicare. http://files.kff.org/attachment/issue-brief-an-overview-of-medicare. Published November 2017. Accessed April 18, 2018.

Kwolek K. Managing MACRA—Part I: What is MACRA? Healthcare Law Insights. http://www.healthcarelawinsights.com/2016/10/managing-macra-part-i-what-is-macra/. Published October 17, 2016. Accessed April 18, 2018.

QualityNet. Fiscal Years 2018–2023 Measures: Hospital Value-Based Purchasing. https://www.qualitynet.org/dcs/ContentServer?c=Page&pagename=QnetPublic%2FPage%2FQnetTier3&cid=1228775522697. Accessed April 18, 2018.

QualityNet. Measures: Hospital-Acquired Condition (HAC) Reduction Program. https://www.qualitynet.org/dcs/ContentServer?c=Page&pagename=QnetPublic%2FPage%2FQnetTier3&cid=1228774294977. Accessed April 18, 2018.

Shafrin J. What Is MACRA? Healthcare Economist. http://healthcare-economist.com/2015/11/01/what-is-macra/. Published November 1, 2015. Accessed April 18, 2018.

2

Primer on Health Plans
Private Insurance

Christopher A. Clyne, MD, MBA
Britton Jewell, DO, MHA

In addition to Medicare and Medicaid (see Chapter 1), private insurance will be the other largest payer source you will encounter. As discussed in Chapter 1, private insurers also deliver Medicare through Part C—Medicare Advantage plans and may also deliver Medicaid through managed care plan arrangements with states. This chapter discusses the different types of private insurance arrangements, the biggest insurance players in the U.S. health care system, and how they reimburse hospitals and providers.

HISTORY OF PRIVATE INSURANCE

The development of organized health insurance, including the concept of deducting a sum of an employee's salary to guarantee health care coverage, can be credited to the railroads in the Western United States in the late 1800s. This practice was also adopted by other industries (eg, mining, lumber, steel, and textiles) to attract and retain employees. By 1930, over half of a million workers were covered by payroll-deducted health plans run by private employers.

In the wake of the Great Depression of 1929, and based on the realization that the average American could not afford the cost of medical care, Superintendent Justin Ford Kimball offered Dallas schoolteachers a hospitalization plan: for 50 cents per month deducted from their pay, each participant would be guaranteed 2 weeks of paid hospital care at Baylor University Hospital. This innovative arrangement of prepayment for health care between Dallas schoolteachers and Baylor University Hospital in 1929 would become BlueCross and BlueShield of Texas—a model for future American health care.

In 1937, the American Hospital Association adopted a plan for group hospitalization with specified standards. This plan was termed "the Blue Cross plan." The public need for a health plan to pay for doctor services was organized by the American Medical Association in 1946 and was dubbed "the Blue Shield plan." These plans were established to provide affordable health care to millions of Americans and offered a viable alternative to compulsory government-controlled health care. These plans served as models for future private health care plans.

Today, 91% of all Americans (over 290 million individuals) are covered by some type of health care plan. Most (56%) have private health care, with the vast majority of these (49% of total) provided under their employer's coverage.

HOW HEALTH PLANS WORK

Health care plans may vary depending on the insurer, but the basic concept is that individuals, or a group of individuals, agree to pay a monthly (annual) fee in exchange for a variety of benefits:

- Doctor's visits
- Prescriptions
- Hospital charges
- Laboratory tests
- Radiology exams
- Emergency room visits
- Home services
- Visiting nurses
- Rehabilitation services
- Behavioral health services
- Addiction services
- Dental services
- Eye care
- Preventive care

Monthly payments (termed premiums) may vary according to age, geographic area, individual group policy, family size, and tobacco use. The Affordable Care Act (ACA), passed by Congress in 2010, eliminated cost adjustments based on gender and preexisting conditions. Plans are offered by a variety of public and private agencies and are purchased generally once per year in marketplaces called "exchanges." Plans are typically tiered on the basis of the amount of monthly premium, copayment, deductible, coinsurance, or maximum out-of-pocket payment that the individual chooses:

- Low monthly premium cost/high deductible
- High monthly premium cost/low deductible

Definitions:

1. Premium—Monthly payment amount

2. Deductible—Amount you pay before insurance coverage begins
3. Copay—Percentage of covered medical services that the individual is responsible for paying
4. Maximum out-of-pocket—The most money an individual or family will pay in 1 year
5. Claims—A doctor or health care facility that performs a service will submit a "claim" for payment to an insurance organization
6. Network—A partnership of local hospitals with physicians and other providers that provide inpatient and outpatient medical and health services to participants in the plan (enrollees). The provider group is paid a set amount per patient enrollee per month. Network physicians may be employees of the network organization (eg, health maintenance organization [HMO], hospital, university) or contracted independent physicians/groups.
7. Health insurance exchanges—Marketplaces where consumers may compare and purchase individual health plans.

TYPES OF PRIVATE INSURANCE

Table 2-1 provides a list of the types of private insurance discussed in this chapter.

MANAGED CARE PLANS

Preferred Provider Organization (PPO)

A type of plan that allows the individual the freedom to choose from a variety of doctors and hospitals in and out of network. Specialists may be seen without preauthorization from the primary care provider. Fees are generally lower for doctors and hospitals in-network than out of network. Providers are part of a plan's network because they are guaranteed patient volume and payment. They have agreed to see patients covered by that insurance plan, and they have agreed to accept the

Table 2-1   Types of Private Insurance

PPO
HMO
Fee-for-service or Indemnity
Point-of-service
Obamacare
Catastrophic coverage

Abbreviations: HMO, health maintenance organization; PPO, preferred provider organization.

health plan's contracted rate, which helps keep coverage affordable. The preferred provider organization (PPO) offers more flexibility and choice for the individual, but at a higher cost compared to an HMO.

Health Maintenance Organization (HMO)

The enrollee's health care is coordinated by a primary care physician who must provide a referral in order for an individual to see a specialist. All doctors and hospital services must be within the network to be covered by the plan. Fees for individuals are generally lower than those of a PPO. Doctors and hospitals benefit from participating in the HMO by enjoying a "guaranteed" large volume of covered patients, and patients benefit by paying lower fees and having access to coordinated services.

Fee-for-Service or Indemnity Plan

These plans are set up to reimburse medical providers for each service the individual receives on a case-by-case basis. Fee-for-service plans allow the choice of any medical provider for health care treatment. Following treatment, the enrollee pays the bill and then sends a claim to the insurer for reimbursement. The insurer may not reimburse 100% for the service. The individual is responsible for the uncovered cost. Indemnity Plan Basics:

- This plan offers the largest choice of doctors, specialists, hospitals, or clinics.
- It does not require a referral or preapproval.
- They can be very expensive, with high premiums and deductibles.
- The plan may not offer coverage for preventive care, so the enrollee might have to pay entirely out of pocket for routine office visits, checkups, vaccinations, etc.
- The plan will reimburse the enrollee only for "covered" medical expenses.
- Typically, indemnity policies have an out-of-pocket maximum. This means that once the covered expenses reach a certain amount in a given calendar year, the insurer will pay the usual and customary fee in full.

Point-of-Service (POS) Plans

A point-of-service (POS) plan is like a hybrid of an HMO and a PPO. The insured can choose to either have a general practitioner coordinate their care or go directly to the "POS" provider.

When the insured requires medical care, there are usually two or three different choices, and they depend on what type of POS plan is in place:

- **Through a primary care physician**—similar to an HMO plan. The insured is just required to make a copayment.
- **PPO network provider services**—the insured can receive care from a PPO provider that is within the PPO's network. The insured will have to

make a copayment and may also be liable for coinsurance (eg, the insurer pays 80% of the bill and the insured the remaining 20%).

- **Services from nonnetwork providers**—some of the medical expenses will be reimbursed. It is important that the insured reads the plan's benefit summary carefully, where who pays for what, and how much, should be clearly laid out. There will usually be a copayment and a higher coinsurance charge.

Government-Sponsored Health Plans (The Affordable Care Act of 2010: Obamacare)

The ACA was designed to provide health insurance to the millions of uninsured Americans at an affordable cost. Coverage options are available from a menu of "metal" options: Platinum, Gold, Silver, and Bronze. The law as written in 2010 provided for a penalty for those who were eligible for insurance but remained uninsured—otherwise known as the "Mandate." This part of the ACA was challenged in court. In 2017 the U.S Supreme Court upheld the Mandate, but President Trump defunded this part of the ACA through the tax/spending bill signed into law on December 22, 2017, thereby jeopardizing the ACA's future.

The plans were created by the ACA to provide essential health benefits to individuals:

- Ambulatory patient services
- Emergency care
- Hospitalization
- Maternity and newborn services
- Mental health and addiction services
- Prescription drug coverage
- Rehabilitative and habilitative care
- Laboratory services
- Preventive and wellness services, along with chronic disease management
- Pediatric care, including dental and vision services

There are four types of "metal" plans based on the amount of coverage versus "out-of-pocket" monthly premium and deductible costs (Figure 2-1).

Catastrophic Health Plan

Catastrophic health insurance plans are available for those under 30 years of age. These plans have low monthly premiums and a very high deductible. They may be an affordable way to protect one's self from worst-case scenarios, such as getting seriously sick or injured. You pay most routine medical expenses yourself. There are no subsidies or tax penalties. Under Obamacare, three primary care visits per year are covered.

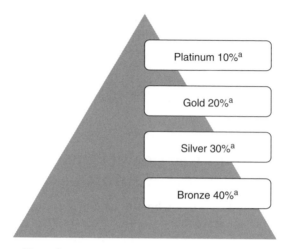

Figure 2-1 Types of "metal" coverage plans with out-of-pocket monthly premium and deductible costs. [a] This percentage refers to the amount the enrollee is expected to cover, which includes the out-of-pocket monthly premium and deductibles; the rest is covered by the insurance plan.

BIGGEST INSURANCE PLAYERS

Table 2-2 lists the largest players in the health insurance industry.

The following are six of the biggest health insurance companies:

- WellPoint
- Cigna
- Aetna
- Humana
- UnitedHealthcare
- BlueCross BlueShield (works on a state-by-state basis)

These six biggest health insurance companies insure approximately half of the insured population, or well over 100 million people. Most major health insurance companies also participate in Medicare Advantage and Obamacare. Medicare Advantage is a plan for Medicare recipients where Medicare (under the Centers for Medicare & Medicaid Services) pays the private insurance company to provide the "same or better" health care coverage for those Medicare recipients who choose to participate.

Table 2-2   Largest Health Insurance Companies

WellPoint	Cigna	Aetna	Humana	UnitedHealthcare	BlueCross BlueShield[a]

[a]Works on a state-by-state basis.

The "Advantage:"

- For individuals is that they receive expanded coverage (eg, vision, dental, hearing, health, and wellness) from a private insurer with a small monthly premium.
- For insurers is that they have a large guaranteed (and growing) population of insured and guaranteed payment by both the government (for administration) and from the individual (for additional services beyond Medicare coverage).
- For the government is that they can reduce labor and administrative costs.

THE FUTURE OF OBAMACARE?

Obamacare is the unofficial name for The Patient Protection and Affordable Care Act (ACA), a health reform law signed on March 23, 2010. The goal of the ACA was to provide health coverage for all children, adults, and families who were uninsured by offering new benefits and rights that were protected by the law.

The ACA offers coverage to millions of Americans who were uninsured by expanding Medicaid in states and in Washington, D.C. who opted to accept federal funding for the expansion. It requires all adults who are eligible to purchase health care through established marketplaces called "exchanges" (found through HealthCare.gov). It established government subsidies for those who could not afford to purchase insurance. It created penalties for those who could afford it but opted not to participate in the exchanges—the "Individual Mandate" (which has since been repealed by the Trump Administration). It established new taxes and tax breaks to pay for the expansion. In 2018 the State of Virginia voted to "opt in" for Medicaid expansion and to provide Obamacare to over 400,000 uninsured. It expanded employer coverage to millions and improved Medicare for seniors and the disabled.

By 2017, 31 states and Washington, DC had opted to expand Medicaid coverage for their citizens, whereas 19 did not. Some insurers ceased providing coverage in 2017 for individuals who were enrolled in Obamacare because of poor revenue performance. Reasons posited for poor revenue included:

- Not enough young, healthy patients with low health care requirements (cost) to offset the overabundance of older patients with preexisting chronic illnesses (many of whom were previously refused coverage) who require high-intensity/cost health care.
- Prices were determined based on erroneous assumptions of "how many" and "who would participate" without any historical data. Many companies priced plans so low that they could not compete in the market.
- Some government subsidies for insurers ended in 2017, resulting in increased operating cost.
- Poor planning and administration—companies experienced in serving Medicaid populations have done well (eg, Kaiser Permanente), whereas

those with experience limited to employer provided plans have struggled (eg, Aetna, UnitedHealthcare).

The future of health care policy is in question following the 2016 Presidential election. President Trump has made it a priority to dismantle the ACA. At the time of this publication, a complete replacement for the ACA has not yet been accepted by Congress or the American public.

Recommended Resources

Badger D. Obamacare's taxpayer-subsidized failure. *National Review*. http://www.national-review.com/article/434546/obamacares-taxpayer-subsidized-failure. Published April 26, 2016. Accessed July 7, 2017.

Baltazar A. The big five: health insurance companies. verywell.com. https://www.verywell.com/the-big-five-health-insurance-companies-2663838. Updated June 25, 2017. Accessed July 7, 2017.

Centers for Medicare & Medicaid Services. Affordable care act. Medicaid.gov. https://www.medicaid.gov/affordable-care-act/index.html. Accessed July 7, 2017.

Centers for Medicare & Medicaid Services. The 'metal' categories: bronze, silver, gold & platinum. HealthCare.gov. https://www.healthcare.gov/choose-a-plan/plans-categories. Accessed July 7, 2017.

Cohn J. Why some Obamacare insurers are making money, but many are losing big. *HuffPost*. http://www.huffingtonpost.com/entry/obamacare-health-insurance_us_573a00dce-4b060aa781ad6cc. Published May 16, 2016. Accessed July 7, 2017.

Kaiser Family Foundation. Health insurance coverage of the total population. http://kff.org/other/state-indicator/total-population. Accessed July 7, 2017.

Obamacare Facts. Types of health insurance plans. http://obamacarefacts.com/insurance-exchange/health-insurance-plans. Accessed July 7, 2017.

Parent to Parent of Georgia. Types of private health insurance plans—the basics. http://roadmap.p2pga.org/index.php/healthcare-59/112-privatehealth-insurance/590-types-of-private-insurance-plans. Accessed July 7, 2017.

3

Physician Reimbursement
How Doctors Are Paid

Christopher A. Clyne, MD, MBA
Britton Jewell, DO, MHA

Few of us who have chosen to be health care professionals have a strong background in finance, but we understand the basic concept that you must make a steady and reasonable salary to pay off your sizable loans, and provide for you and your family.

The equation seems simple, but here are important variables that can result in great disappointment and jeopardize compensation (and even employment) if not fully understood before entering into an employment situation. It is imperative that the employment candidate understand the compensation models before agreeing to a contract, even as health care reform is changing these models. The goal of this chapter is to help the practitioner understand the various payment models that will affect his or her income and future.

TYPES OF PAYMENT MODELS

Fee-for-Service

This is perhaps the easiest payment model to comprehend: health care providers are paid for the services that they provide. These may include office visits, medical tests, procedures, and operations (Figure 3-1).

Supporters argue that the positives include a simpler understanding of the transaction between a provider and the patient. Some claim that this payment model encourages competition and results in a higher productivity of incentivized providers. Detractors of this model argue that it encourages unnecessary visits and procedures,

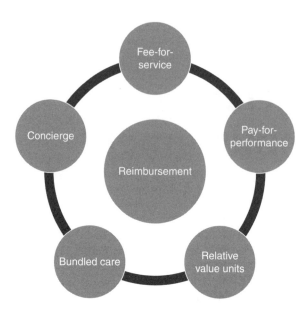

Figure 3-1 Types of physician payment models.

thus inflating the cost of health care without an improvement in quality. Further, it is claimed that health care is delivered in an itinerant manner rather than in an integrated holistic approach—fixing what is wrong rather than preventing illness.

Fee-for-service has been the subject of discussion and motivation for change since the 1990s because health care costs were rising at an accelerated rate of more than 10% of gross domestic product (GDP) and continued to rise to almost 18% of GDP in 2018 (Table 3-1).

Performance-Based Payment

The U.S. economy is a private economy. It is also (in theory) a meritocracy, where workers can advance based on their performance and value to the company.

Performance-based compensation is seen in many industries familiar to us: chief executive officers and stockholders alike are "bonused" when their company's performance (stock value) is good. Professional athletes are bonused when they reach the final playoffs. Workers who advance in a company owing to their accomplishments are typically rewarded with a higher salary. The goal is to incentivize workers and executives to perform at a higher level, thus benefiting themselves and the organization.

Pay-for-performance (P4P), or value-based purchasing, in medicine is a payment model that offers financial incentives to physicians, hospitals, nursing homes, and other health care providers for meeting certain quality metrics.

The following were some of the most influential performance-based programs that have been rolled into the Medicare Access and CHIP Reauthorization Act (MACRA) of 2015 and repackaged as the Merit-Based Incentive Payment System (MIPS), which ties the Centers for Medicare & Medicaid Services' (CMS)

TABLE 3-1 Total Expenditure on Health as a Share of GDP

	1970	1980	1990	2000	2008
Australia	4.1%[d]	6.1%	6.7%	8.0%	8.5%[d]
Austria	5.2%	7.4%	8.3%[a]	9.9%	10.5%
Belgium	3.9%	6.3%	7.2%	9.0%[b,c]	11.1%[b,c]
Canada	6.9%	7.0%	8.9%	8.8%	10.4%[c]
France	5.4%	7.0%	8.4%	10.1%	11.2%
Germany	N/A	N/A	N/A	10.3%	10.5%
Italy	N/A	N/A	7.7%	8.1%	9.1%
Japan	4.6%	6.5%	6.0%	7.7%	8.1%[d]
Netherlands	N/A	7.4%	8.0%	8.0%	9.9%[c]
Norway	4.4%	7.0%	7.6%	8.4%	8.5%[c]
Spain	3.5%	5.3%	6.5%	7.2%	9.0%
Sweden	6.8%	8.9%	8.2%	8.2%	9.4%
Switzerland	5.4%	7.3%	8.2%	10.2%	10.7%[c]
United Kingdom	4.5%	5.6%	5.9%	7.0%	8.7%
United States	7.1%	9.0%	12.2%	13.4%	16.0%
Average	5.2%	7.0%	7.8%	9.0%	10.1%

[a]Break in series.
[b]Differences in methodology.
[c]Estimate.
[d]Estimate from prior calendar year.
Abbreviations: GDP, gross domestic product; N/A, not applicable.
Kaiser Family Foundation. Snapshots: health care spending in the United States & selected OECD countries. http://kff.org/health-costs/issue-brief/snapshots-health-care-spending-in-the-united-states-selected-oecd-countries. Published April 12, 2011. Accessed July 7, 2017.

payments to performance on the basis of four dimensions: clinical quality, resource use, health IT meaningful use, and clinical practice improvement activities.

1. Hospital Value-Based Purchasing Program. This program rewards acute care hospitals with incentive payments for the quality of care they give to people with Medicare. It withholds payments to participating hospitals by a specified percentage and uses those funds for the bonus payments. The rewards are granted based on how well the hospital performs on 20 quality measures. For each measure, the hospital earns a score for achievement and for improvement. The better the hospital's overall score, the more it receives in bonus payments. Acute care hospitals account for the largest share of Medicare spending, and the program reaches over 3,500 hospitals across the country.

2. Hospital Readmission Reduction Program. This program provides financial incentives to hospitals to reduce unnecessary hospital readmissions (not including planned readmissions) that are costly and usually due to a lack of coordination between providers, inadequate discharge planning, and poor follow-up with patients. The program can reduce payments by 1% for hospitals that exceed certain readmission rates for patients with acute myocardial infarction (AMI), heart failure, pneumonia, chronic obstructive pulmonary disease (COPD), elective total hip and/or total knee replacement, and coronary artery bypass graft (CABG) surgery.

3. Physician Value Modifier Program. This program rewards physicians with bonus payments when their performance attains specified measures of quality and cost. The adjustments are made on a per claim basis for items and services under the Medicare Physician Fee Schedule. CMS is phasing in the program, beginning with physicians' groups with 100 or more eligible professionals in 2015 and extending the value modifier to all physicians and most health care practitioners (eg, physician assistants and nurse specialists) by 2018.

4. Physician Quality Reporting System. This program incentivizes physicians and group practices to report information to Medicare about the quality of their services. In 2015, the program began applying a negative payment adjustment to physicians and practice groups who did not report data on the quality measures specified in the program.[1]

The triumvirate goals of modern health care are to improve safety, reduce cost/improve efficiency, and improve quality outcomes. The P4P model rewards providers, hospitals, and organizations for meeting these goals and penalizes those who do not. Examples of efforts to improve safety include targeting of hospital-acquired conditions (HACs), provider-preventable conditions, and health care–associated infections: These include preventable falls, catheter-based infections, and prescribing errors. CMS estimates that approximately 50 000 fewer patients died in the hospital as a result of a reduction in HACs, and approximately $12 billion in health care costs was saved from 2010 through 2013 through these efforts.

Many of the practices of CMS have been adopted by private insurers. Performance is evaluated by analyzing claims and administrative data, which require some documentation addressing four main areas:

- **Process improvement**—for example, documentation that patients who smoke were counseled to quit and were given alternatives.
- **Outcomes measurement**—for example, reduction in readmission rates for congestive heart failure and COPD patients.
- **Infrastructure improvements**—for example, implementation of electronic health records.
- **Patient satisfaction**—for example, reduced waiting times and improved patient–doctor communication.

Relative Value Units Payment System

Most physicians are reimbursed as a combination of a base salary and productivity measured in relative value units (RVUs). The RVU system was introduced in 1992 by CMS as a way of reducing cost and standardizing physician compensation among the variety of specialties, services, and procedures. A work RVU was created for each of the thousands of services and procedures found in the Physician Fee Schedule.

The dollar amount for each service or procedure (assigned a current procedural terminology [CPT] code copyrighted by the American Medical Association) was determined by physician's work, practice expenses, and malpractice insurance (with a geographic multiplier). This formula was felt to account for services and procedures requiring additional (specialist) training, expense, and risk.

The upside of this payment system is that physicians and other providers are compensated based on the complexity of the task and their training. Further, it encourages efficiency and productivity. The downside is that it may encourage the physician to see more patients by spending, perhaps, less time per patient in nonreimbursable tasks like education.

The RVU system has some features of a fee-for-service model of payment: procedure-based specialties are reimbursed more aggressively than primary care or pediatrics. This may encourage performance of procedures and tests instead of less complex but time-consuming record retrieval or history taking of family members. Additionally, this system may discourage the provider from seeing high-risk patients or those requiring procedures of lesser revenue-based value.

Despite its flaws, the RVU system has become the national standard for all insurers. Physician contracts, hospital contracts, and industry contracts will all be impacted by the RVU system. It is important for providers, administrators, and health care–related groups to understand the complexities and vagaries of this system of reimbursement.

Bundled Care Models

The bundled care model is a scion of the capitated care model of the 1990s. In the capitated care model, health care payment model providers were paid a fixed amount per patient per time period, regardless of use. The amount was determined by the individual patient characteristics and risk. There was a financial incentive to deliver care at reduced cost, less than the amount paid by the insurer. Health care providers then had an incentive to keep patients healthy in order to avoid high-cost procedures and hospitalizations. There was also an incentive to exclude high-risk patients or to avoid potentially helpful tests/procedures if "over-budget." As the populations of young healthy enrollees from the 1990s aged into a higher-risk, costlier demographic, health maintenance organizations, and their providers realized that the model needed revision.

Bundled care refers to a fixed payment by the insurer for a single episode of care to multiple providers (eg, hospital and physicians) for all related services (eg, preop, surgery, postop care). This method of payment encourages alignment and efficiency among providers although not discouraging providers from caring for more complex, high-risk patients. Disadvantages include the potential incentive for "cherry-picking" procedures and patients and limiting access to specialists and more expensive procedures/tests. There are several versions of "bundling" based on different risk-sharing options and types of procedures.

Retainer (Concierge) Medicine

This model of practice is discussed in the "Practice Paradigms" section. It is mentioned in this chapter on physician payment because it presents the individual practitioner with a practice and payment model that is a hybrid of a fee-for-service model and a contracted, or retainer, model.

It works like this: the patient pays a monthly or yearly retainer in cash directly for the services of a doctor, usually a primary care provider, avoiding the insurance company. The doctor (or small practice) limits the number of patients in his or her practice, allowing each provider to dedicate more time and attention to each patient. It is also called "enhanced care" because the arrangement typically involves unfettered and immediate access to the physician(s).

Practice models can differ, as do the fees: under $100 per month to thousands annually. Most practice arrangements cover unlimited office visits and communications with the provider by phone, text, video, or e-mail without a copay. There may be an additional cash fee for special tests, immunizations, and procedures (fee-for-care).

Many concierge practices also accept nonretainer patients and charge an additional fee to provide services not covered by insurance or Medicare. This hybrid model—fee-for-extra care—permits the practice a broader patient base and an opportunity to enhance income, while providing patients with "full service" without the burden of full payment.

Most concierge practices limit their practices to "cash-only" patients. This reduces overhead and administrative cost, improves efficiency, and allows for more time per patient. It also provides an enhanced income for the primary practice provider, similar to the specialists' income.

HOW MUCH COMPENSATION CAN I EXPECT AFTER RESIDENCY?

Salary is what most new/new-to-practice physicians and providers focus on when considering a job. There are other very important components of employment as a physician or health care professional to consider during the negotiations. Take time to consider and investigate these:

- Call schedule—Time away from family. Extra hours usually at night and on weekends. How frequent?
- Colleagues—How many? Collaborative or competitive? Do they value continuing education or is it just another distraction? Is there a pecking order (seniors don't take calls)?
- How many practice sites are you responsible for (eg, hospitals, surgery centers, offices, labs, clinics)?
- How long to partnership if in practice? Is there a "buy in"?

- "At will" or protected? Can you be "let go" without cause at the discretion of the employer? Is there a severance arrangement?
- Continuing medical education support—days and dollars—how many/how much?
- Performance review process—by whom, how often, what are the metrics? Does future compensation depend on these reviews?
- Noncompete clause—how far and how long? Is it enforceable in that state?
- Tail coverage—does the insurance policy cover a "tail" if you leave the practice? Otherwise, you must cover the cost of a "tail."

Salary is important. It undoubtedly influenced (to some degree) your decision to enter medicine/health care and choose a specialty within health care. The self-reported 2016 incomes of some 19 200 physicians across 27 specialties as reported by Web-MD in Medscape's 2017 Physician Compensation Report is presented in Table 3-2.

TABLE 3-2   How Much Money Physicians Make

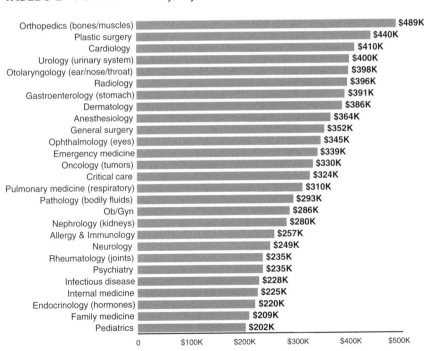

Orthopedics (bones/muscles)	$489K
Plastic surgery	$440K
Cardiology	$410K
Urology (urinary system)	$400K
Otolaryngology (ear/nose/throat)	$398K
Radiology	$396K
Gastroenterology (stomach)	$391K
Dermatology	$386K
Anesthesiology	$364K
General surgery	$352K
Ophthalmology (eyes)	$345K
Emergency medicine	$339K
Oncology (tumors)	$330K
Critical care	$324K
Pulmonary medicine (respiratory)	$310K
Pathology (bodily fluids)	$293K
Ob/Gyn	$286K
Nephrology (kidneys)	$280K
Allergy & Immunology	$257K
Neurology	$249K
Rheumatology (joints)	$235K
Psychiatry	$235K
Infectious disease	$228K
Internal medicine	$225K
Endocrinology (hormones)	$220K
Family medicine	$209K
Pediatrics	$202K

Grisham S. Medscape physician compensation report 2017. Medscape. http://www.medscape.com/slideshow/compensation-2017-overview-6008547?src=wnl_physrep_170405_mscpmrk_comp2017&uac=14967FJ&impID=1322713&faf=1#4. Published April 5, 2017. Accessed July 7, 2017.

CONCLUSION

Understanding payment models is an important requisite for choosing a job and understanding how you will be paid. Understanding how you get paid will influence your decision to join a small or large practice, be an employed or independent physician or be a primary care physician or a specialist.

Although salary is a big part of the compensation package, it is not the only thing to consider when choosing a specialty, a job, or perhaps a different practice model (see Chapter 13). Take time to consider the less obvious, yet critically important, aspects of the compensation package, including the employer's/institution's commitment to you and your responsibilities to the employer/institution.

Reference

1. Baird C. Top healthcare stories for 2016: pay-for-performance. Committee for Economic Development. https://www.ced.org/blog/entry/top-healthcare-stories-for-2016-pay-for-performance. Published March 8, 2016. Accessed July 7, 2017.

Recommended Resources

Agency for Healthcare Research and Quality. 2013 Annual hospital-acquired condition rate and estimates of cost savings and deaths averted from 2010 to 2013. http://www.ahrq.gov/professionals/quality-patient-safety/pfp/hacrate2013.html. Published October, 2015. Accessed July 7, 2017.

American Association for Marriage and Family Therapy. Private payer summary. https://www.aamft.org/iMIS15/AAMFT/Content/Advocacy/Private_Payer_Summary.aspx. Accessed July 7, 2017.

Bendix J. RVUs: a valuable tool for aiding practice management. Medical Economics. http://www.medicaleconomics.com/health-law-policy/rvus-valuable-tool-aiding-practice-management. Published February 25, 2014. Accessed July 7, 2017.

Bundled payments for care improvement (BPCI) initiative: general information. CMS.gov. https://innovation.cms.gov/initiatives/bundled-payments. Updated July 5, 2017. Accessed July 7, 2017.

Concierge Medicine Today. 2012–2015 Concierge physician salary report. https://conciergemedicinetoday.org/2014-concierge-physician-salary-report. Published September 9, 2015. Accessed July 7, 2017.

Evans M. U.S. officials finalize rule for Medicare payments to doctors. The Wall Street Journal. https://www.wsj.com/articles/u-s-officials-finalize-rule-for-medicare-payments-to-doctors-1476466755. Published October 14, 2016. Accessed July 7, 2017.

Federal Register. Medicare Program; Revisions to Payment Policies Under the Physician Fee Schedule and Other Revisions to Part B for CY 2017; Medicare Advantage Bid Pricing Data Release; Medicare Advantage and Part D Medical Loss Ratio Data Release; Medicare Advantage Provider Network Requirements; Expansion of Medicare Diabetes Prevention Program Model; Medicare Shared Savings Program Requirements. https://www.federalregister.gov/documents/2016/11/15/2016-26668/medicare-program-revisions-to-payment-policies-under-the-physician-fee-schedule-and-other-revisions. Published November 15, 2016. Accessed July 7, 2017.

Grisham S. Medscape physician compensation report 2017. Medscape. http://www
.medscape.com/slideshow/compensation-2017-overview-6008547?src=wnl_
physrep_170405_mscpmrk_comp2017&uac=14967FJ&impID=1322713&faf=1#4.
Published April 5, 2017. Accessed July 7, 2017.

Japsen B. How the White House changes doctors' Medicare pay in 2,398 pages. *Forbes.* http://
www.forbes.com/sites/brucejapsen/2016/10/15/how-the-white-house-is-changing-
doctor-medicare-pay-in-2398-pages/#5be65c2c281d. Published October 15, 2016.
Accessed July 7, 2017.

Kaiser Family Foundation. Snapshots: health care spending in the United States & selected
OECD countries. http://kff.org/health-costs/issue-brief/snapshots-health-care-
spending-in-the-united-states-selected-oecd-countries. Published April 12, 2011.
Accessed July 7, 2017.

Reed LS. Private health insurance in the United States: an overview. Social Security
Administration. https://www.ssa.gov/policy/docs/ssb/v28n12/v28n12p3.pdf. Published
December, 1965. Accessed July 7, 2017.

4

Nonprofit or Not
How Hospitals Are Paid

Christopher A. Clyne, MD, MBA
Britton Jewell, DO, MHA

In Chapter 1, we discussed the major payers in the U.S. health care system, Medicare and Medicaid. Additionally, in Chapter 2, we discussed private insurers. This chapter addresses the question of how these payers reimburse hospitals as well as additional ways hospitals receive funds.

Medicare payment rates are set by the federal government, and Medicaid payment rates are set by state governments. Private insurance companies negotiate directly with the hospitals to set the payment rates. Uninsured patients or those outside their insurance policy network are billed directly by the hospital.

Because these payment rates are set by the payers themselves, they don't always cover the hospital's actual cost of providing care. Medicare and Medicaid payment rates are set low, which, according to the American Hospital Association, results in billions of dollars of *underreimbursed* care. "Underpayment by Medicare and Medicaid to U.S. hospitals was $57.8 billion in 2015."[1]

The hospital also bears the costs for the free care provided to the uninsured called *uncompensated* care. "Since 2000, hospitals of all types have provided more than $538 billion in *uncompensated* care to their patients."[2]

Therefore, the hospital must rely on private insurance payments in order to recover some costs. The different proportions of the total hospital's reimbursement paid by various sources is termed the *payer mix*. A favorable payer mix would be composed of sources with the highest reimbursements, such as Medicare and private insurers.

For fiscal year 2013, only 45% of U.S. acute care hospitals made a profit. Some factors associated with *increased profitability* include state price regulation, higher prices for services, for-profit standing, and association with a larger health care system. Some factors associated with *decreased profitability* include a larger population of uninsured patients, a larger population of Medicare patients, or location in an area with a high proportion of health maintenance organization patients and/or one main health insurance company.[3]

HOW MEDICARE PAYS HOSPITALS

Hospitals get paid when a Medicare patient is discharged after receiving an episode of inpatient care or comes to the hospital's outpatient department to receive services. As discussed in Chapter 1, Medicare utilizes the Inpatient Prospective Payment System (IPPS) to set reimbursement rates for an episode of inpatient care and the Outpatient Prospective Payment System (OPPS) for outpatient care.

Inpatient Services

How much money the hospital will receive depends primarily on the *discharge diagnosis* of the patient. Medicare sets a base rate of payment based on the Diagnosis-Related Group (DRG) that correlates to the discharge diagnosis. Medical diagnoses can vary widely, but each encounter can be funneled into 1 of over 750 DRGs. The final DRG depends on more than just the primary discharge diagnosis and can be modified by applying up to 24 secondary diagnoses and up to 25 procedures that may have taken place during the hospitalization.

Secondary diagnoses are categorized based on how sick the patient is, termed the *severity of illness*, and how many *health care resources* the patient can be expected to use.

There are three different *severity of illness* categories that are part of the *Medicare Severity (MS)–DRG program*, and they are termed Major Complication/Comorbidity (MCC), Complication/Comorbidity (CC), and Non–Complication/Comorbidity (non-CC). A higher severity of illness will result in a DRG with a higher reimbursement rate. It is critically important to document each patient's primary diagnosis and all comorbidities that were present during the episode of care (eg, acute kidney injury, diabetes mellitus, hypokalemia, cardiac arrest) for optimal reimbursement.

The total base reimbursement rate is calculated based on the combined contribution of two separate cost centers: *operating costs* and *capital costs*.

Operating costs are those costs incurred in the operation of the hospital itself and include labor, utilities, and the purchase of disposable equipment—generally, the cost of daily operations. *Capital costs* are associated with maintaining the property, property acquisitions and improvements, fixed and movable equipment (eg, magnetic resonance imaging scanners), the building, building fixtures, and improvements.

The total base rate then undergoes several modifications to arrive at the final amount. The MS–DRG is assigned a final weight based on these factors. An additional modification is made based on geographic wage variations throughout the country. Hospitals can receive additional payments from Medicare if they have a residency program, if they treat a high proportion of low-income patients (termed *disproportionate share hospital* [DSH]), and if they have any exceptionally complicated and high-cost cases (termed *high case mix index*). Medicare will also reimburse a hospital's *unreimbursed care* (called bad debt) at 65% if it remains unpaid after it has been sent to collections.

HOW QUALITY IS TIED TO REIMBURSEMENT

Hospitals may be *penalized and receive reduced payments from Medicare* if they have excessive readmissions *within 30 days of discharge* for certain diagnoses, including (see complete list in the "Hospital Readmissions Reduction Program" section):

- Acute myocardial infarction (AMI)
- Congestive heart failure (HF)
- Pneumonia (PN)

under the Hospital Readmissions Reduction Program (HRRP); if they do not perform well in certain quality measures under the Hospital Value-Based Purchasing (VBP) Program; and/or if they are in the bottom 25% for certain hospital-acquired conditions (HACs) under the HAC Reduction Program such as the following:

- Central line and surgical site infections
- Methicillin-resistant *Staphylococcus aureus* (MRSA) bacteremia
- *Clostridium difficile* infections (CDI)
- Patient safety scores (Patient Safety Indicator [PSI] 90 composite score)

Figure 4-1 provides a summary of all of Medicare's quality improvement programs that affect a hospital's reimbursement. All of these programs are discussed in detail in a subsequent section.

Hospital Value-Based Purchasing Program

The Hospital VBP Program ties quality measures to reimbursement. This program "justifies" a reduction in the overall DRG payments to a hospital by providing *value-based incentive payments* to those hospitals that perform well in the following *quality areas*:

- Care coordination and patient experience
- Clinical processes and outcomes

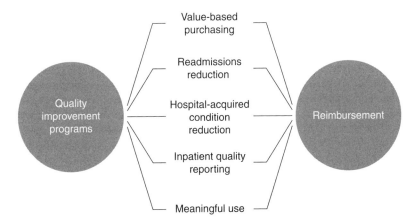

Figure 4-1 Medicare programs that tie quality to reimbursement.

- Lowering costs and improving efficiency
- Patient safety

In the current legislation, there is a 2% reduction in the base Centers for Medicare & Medicaid Services (CMS) payment for every DRG. Quality measures within the *quality areas* listed earlier are combined to produce a *Total Performance Score (TPS)*. These quality measures are recorded in the electronic health record (EHR) and standardized survey sites. The hospitals that perform well receive value-based incentive payments that are funded through the 2% base reductions.

The performance measures that are tied to reimbursement are as follows:

- Fibrinolytic medication for AMI patients within 30 minutes
- Influenza vaccination for patients aged 6 months and older
- Number of unnecessary scheduled deliveries for pregnancy before 39 weeks
- Mortality rates for HF, AMI, and PN
- Agency for Healthcare Research and Quality (AHRQ) PSI 90 Composite (described in detail in a subsequent section)
- Centers for Disease Control and Prevention (CDC) National Healthcare Safety Network (NHSN) Healthcare-Associated Infection (HAI) measures (described in detail in a subsequent section)
- Amount of spending per Medicare patient
- Hospital Consumer Assessment of Healthcare Providers and Systems (HCAHPS) survey scores (patient satisfaction)

The **HCAHPS** scores, also known as "patient satisfaction" scores, make up the Care Coordination and Patient Experience domain of the VBP program and account for *25% of the TPS*. The HCAHPS survey was created by CMS and the AHRQ and is administered either by the hospitals themselves or through an approved third-party surveyor. It is composed of 32 questions covering multiple areas of a patient's experience in the hospital, such as doctor and nurse communication, pain management, and discharge information. For a sample survey, see https://www.hcahpsonline.org/globalassets/hcahps/survey-instruments/mail/july-1-2018-and-forward-discharges/2018_survey-instruments_english_mail.pdf.

Hospital Readmissions Reduction Program

The Hospital Readmissions Reduction Program reduces overall payments by up to 3% to hospitals with readmissions within 30 days for certain conditions. As of 2018, the conditions that are reportable for 30-day readmission penalties included:

- AMI
- HF
- PN
- Acute exacerbation of chronic obstructive pulmonary disease
- Elective total hip arthroplasty
- Elective total knee arthroplasty
- Coronary artery bypass graft surgery

Hospital-Acquired Condition Reduction Program

The HAC Reduction Program decreases overall Medicare payments by 1% for hospitals that perform in the bottom 25% for preventable conditions. A hospital's score is calculated from the data for quality measures that are divided into *two domains*:

Domain 1 is composed of measures that make up the AHRQ PSI 90 Composite. For 2018, the CMS used a Recalibrated PSI 90 Composite score, which included the following measures:

- Pressure ulcer rate
- Iatrogenic pneumothorax rate
- In-hospital fall with hip fracture rate
- Perioperative hemorrhage or hematoma rate
- Postoperative wound dehiscence rate
- Postoperative acute kidney injury requiring dialysis rate
- Postoperative respiratory failure rate
- Perioperative pulmonary embolism or deep vein thrombosis rate
- Postoperative sepsis rate
- Unrecognized abdominopelvic accidental puncture/laceration rate

Domain 2 is composed of the CDC NHSN HAI measures. As of 2018, the reportable conditions included:

- Catheter-associated urinary tract infection
- Central line–associated bloodstream infection
- MRSA bacteremia
- CDI
- Surgical site infection for colon and hysterectomy

With these three programs combined, up to 6% of the hospital reimbursement can be affected. It is important to understand that many hospitals survive solely through Medicare reimbursements and maintain slim margins of only a few percent every year. A reduction of even 1% of all the Medicare payments for the year can be devastating for a hospital.

Thus, hospitals are paying attention to these metrics and to the quality of care being provided by their employees. Additionally, the data for all of these programs and other quality measures are published at Medicare's Hospital Compare website at www.medicare.gov/hospitalcompare, where consumers can browse and compare data from thousands of hospitals throughout the nation.

Adjustments to Inpatient Rates

CMS makes a final adjustment to the operating payment rate on an annual basis based on the expected increased cost of providing patient care, termed the *market basket update*. For 2018, this was an increase of 1.2%. For a hospital to receive this increased payment, it must participate in the Hospital Inpatient Quality Reporting (IQR) Program and be a meaningful EHR user.

Hospital Inpatient Quality Reporting Program

The Hospital IQR Program incentivizes hospitals to report their quality measures to CMS in an effort to improve the quality of care for their patients. Starting in 2016, these measures were required to be submitted electronically. The quality measures reported can be compared among hospitals at the Hospital Compare website. Some of these quality measures are already included in the Hospital VBP Program, but the following are among those that are not: the use of the sepsis bundle, venous thromboembolism prophylaxis, and the stroke 30-day readmission rate. Some measures are voluntarily reported, such as beta-blocker use for AMI and prophylactic antibiotic use for surgical patients. Starting in 2015 and beyond, hospitals that fail to report the required quality measures will see their *market basket update* reduced by one-fourth!

Electronic Health Record (EHR) Incentive Programs

The EHR Incentive Programs promote the meaningful use of EHRs for hospitals and providers. The programs are divided into three stages:

- Stage 1: Created requirements for collection of electronic data and giving patients electronic copies of their data
- Stage 2: Promoted use of EHRs to improve clinical quality and sharing of data
- Stage 3: Promoted use of EHRs to improve health outcomes

Starting in 2017 and beyond, *hospitals* that are not meaningful EHR users will see their market basket update reduced by three-fourths! As a side note, for *health care providers*, the EHR Incentive Programs has been replaced by the Quality Payment Program starting in 2017. The Quality Payment Program establishes the Advanced Alternative Payment Models and the Merit-based Incentive Payment System discussed in detail in Chapter 1.

Table 4-1 summarizes the similarities and differences between these Medicare quality programs.

OUTPATIENT SERVICES

The OPPS covers hospital outpatient services such as:

- Outpatient surgical procedures
- Radiology services
- Hospital clinic or emergency room visits
- Observation admissions
- Some drugs
- Some durable medical equipment

Some inpatient services under Medicare Part B (such as when an inpatient admission that should have been billed as an observation/outpatient is declined by CMS) and partial hospitalization services are reimbursed to hospitals under

TABLE 4-1 Comparison of Medicare Quality Programs

	Value-Based Purchasing	Readmissions Reduction	Hospital-Acquired Condition Reduction	Inpatient Quality Reporting	Meaningful Use
Affect reimbursement	X	X	X	X	X
HCAHPS	X				
AHRQ PSI 90 measures	X		X		
CDC NHSN HAI measures	X		X		
Reportable readmissions		X			
Quality measures	X			X	
EHR use					X

Abbreviations: AHRQ, Agency for Healthcare Research and Quality; CDC, Centers for Disease Control and Prevention; EHR, electronic health record; HAI, Healthcare-Associated Infection; HCAHPS, Hospital Consumer Assessment of Healthcare Providers and System; NHSN, National Healthcare Safety Network; PSI, Patient Safety Indicator.

the OPPS. Partial hospitalization services refer to mental health treatment programs, such as a day program, which takes place in the hospital.

The base reimbursement rate for outpatient services is based on the *Ambulatory Payment Classification (APC)*. The outpatient service delivered, such as minor surgery, which corresponds to a Healthcare Common Procedure Coding System (HCPCS) code, is then ascribed to an APC. For more information regarding the HCPCS, see Chapter 1.

Of note, there are many outpatient services that are reimbursed separately and are not included in an APC bundle. For example, most emergency room visits, most clinic visits, some preventative services, some drugs, some surgical procedures, and partial hospitalization services are reimbursed independently.

The final APC amount is further modified by the local wage rates and the amount of resources consumed by the service. Hospitals may also receive additional payments for high-cost outlier cases if they are a cancer hospital or a children's hospital, or in a rural area.

HOW MEDICAID PAYS HOSPITALS

Medicaid payments are not standardized, but are determined by each state. Inpatient services are reimbursed per DRG in a fee-for-service manner, or in a managed care arrangement. Each state decides the base reimbursement amount, which may be a certain proportion of the Medicare DRG. In addition to this base amount, Medicaid makes supplemental payments to hospitals based on governmental programs, such as waivers. DSH payments are made to hospitals that provide care for a large number of Medicaid enrollees or the poor. Each state may have a different mix of fee-for-service, supplemental payments, and DSH payments made to hospitals. This mix may result in payments that do not cover the entire cost of services provided. Through the Medicaid expansion brought on by the Affordable Care Act (ACA), hospitals are receiving a greater amount of these payments. However, the ACA will start to lower DSH payments by $2 billion in 2018, reducing payments further by $8 billion in 2025. It is unknown how this will affect hospitals' solvency, but it is unlikely that the decrease in DSH payments will be completely offset by the increase in fee-for-service payments resulting from an influx of newly insured Medicaid patients. Safety-net hospitals, which have the highest proportion of Medicaid or uninsured admissions, could be drastically affected by these payment reductions. Outpatient Medicaid services are reimbursed as fee-for-service payments set by each state.

HOW PRIVATE INSURANCE PAYS HOSPITALS

Private insurers negotiate directly with hospitals to determine their fee schedule. These rates are usually deeply discounted and are not the rate the hospital charges. Inpatient and outpatient services are reimbursed in this way. Some insurance companies use the Medicare DRGs and set their own rates for each admission, procedure, and encounter.

UNINSURED PATIENTS

Patients without insurance, termed self-pay, are billed directly by the hospital, typically at a discounted rate. If the debt remains unpaid after a certain period of time, the hospital is able to write it off. Currently, CMS reimburses hospitals 65% of the Medicare payment for unreimbursed care. Some hospitals sell their outstanding debt to collection companies that may resort to legal action to collect payment.

THE TRIUMVIRATE OF HEALTH CARE: QUALITY, SAFETY, AND REDUCED COST

Many hospitals run on extremely thin margins of only a few percent. The payment schema for hospitals is extremely complex and requires an understanding of federal, state, and private insurance practices and policies. It also requires a deep understanding of the cost basis of the institution down to the operating and capital costs of each department and an understanding of the health needs of their local population. Hospitals are meeting these challenges by adopting the principles and practices adopted by CMS and large health care organizations, detailed earlier, in an effort to improve the *quality* and *safety* of health care while ensuring efficient service delivery aimed at reducing *cost.*

The better you understand the financial situation and practices of the health care institution that you are connected to, the better you can assess your future at that institution.

References

1. American Hospital Association. Financial fact sheets. https://www.aha.org/guides-reports/2017-02-11-financial-fact-sheets. Accessed August 19, 2017.
2. American Hospital Association. Uncompensated hospital care cost fact sheet. https://www.aha.org/system/files/2018-01/2017-uncompensated-care-factsheet.pdf. Published December, 2016. Accessed August 19, 2017.
3. Ge B, Anderson GF. A more detailed understanding of factors associated with hospital profitability. *Health Aff.* 2016;35(5):889-897. https://www.healthaffairs.org/doi/abs/10.1377/hlthaff.2015.1193. Accessed August 19, 2017.

Recommended Resources

American Hospital Association. Assistance to low-income Medicare beneficiaries (bad debt). https://www.aha.org/system/files/content/11/110909-baddebt.pdf. Published September 8, 2015. Accessed August 19, 2017.

American Hospital Association. Hospital billing explained. https://www.aha.org/fact-sheet/2015-03-18-hospital-billing-explained. Published March 18, 2015. Accessed August 19, 2017.

American Hospital Association. Underpayment by Medicare and Medicaid fact sheet. https://www.aha.org/system/files/2018-01/medicaremedicaidunderpmt%202017.pdf. Published December 2016. Accessed August 19, 2017.

Centers for Medicare & Medicaid Services. Acute care hospital inpatient prospective payment system. https://www.cms.gov/Outreach-and-Education/Medicare-Learning-Network-MLN/MLNProducts/downloads/AcutePaymtSysfctsht.pdf. Published December 2016. Accessed August 19, 2017.

Centers for Medicare & Medicaid Services. Electronic health records (EHR) incentive programs. https://www.cms.gov/Regulations-and-Guidance/Legislation/EHRIncentivePrograms/index.html. Updated July 13, 3017. Accessed August 19, 2017.

Centers for Medicare & Medicaid Services. Fiscal Year (FY) 2018 Medicare Hospital Inpatient Prospective Payment System (IPPS) and Long Term Acute Care Hospital (LTCH) Prospective Payment System Final Rule (CMS-1677-F). https://www.cms.gov/Newsroom/MediaReleaseDatabase/Fact-sheets/2017-Fact-Sheet-items/2017-08-02.html. Published August 2, 2017. Accessed April 24, 2018.

Centers for Medicare & Medicaid Services. Hospital Inpatient Prospective Payment System (IPPS) and Long Term Acute Care Hospital (LTCH) Final Rule Policy and Payment Changes for Fiscal Year (FY) 2017. https://www.cms.gov/Newsroom/MediaReleaseDatabase/Fact-sheets/2016-Fact-sheets-items/2016-08-02.html. Published August 2, 2016. Accessed August 19, 2017.

Centers for Medicare & Medicaid Services. Hospital outpatient prospective payment system. https://www.cms.gov/Outreach-and-Education/Medicare-Learning-Network-MLN/MLNProducts/downloads/HospitalOutpaysysfctsht.pdf. Published January 2016. Accessed August 19, 2017.

Centers for Medicare & Medicaid Services. Hospital-acquired condition reduction program fiscal year 2018 fact sheet. https://www.cms.gov/Medicare/Medicare-Fee-for-Service-Payment/AcuteInpatientPPS/Downloads/FY2018-HAC-Reduction-Program-Fact-Sheet.pdf. Accessed April 24, 2018.

Centers for Medicare & Medicaid Services. New stratified methodology hospital-level impact file user guide: hospital readmissions reduction program. https://www.cms.gov/Medicare/Medicare-Fee-for-Service-Payment/AcuteInpatientPPS/Downloads/HRRP_StratMethod_ImpctFile_UG.PDF. Published November, 2017. Accessed April 24, 2018.

Cubanski J, Swoope C, Boccuti C, et al. A primer on Medicare: key facts about the Medicare program and the people it covers. Kaiser Family Foundation. http://kff.org/report-section/a-primer-on-medicare-how-does-medicare-pay-providers-in-traditional-medicare/. Published March 20, 2015. Accessed August 19, 2017.

Cunningham P, Rudowitz R, Young K, Garfield R, Foutz J. Understanding Medicaid hospital payments and the impact of recent policy changes. Kaiser Family Foundation. https://www.kff.org/medicaid/issue-brief/understanding-medicaid-hospital-payments-and-the-impact-of-recent-policy-changes/. Published June 8, 2016. Accessed August 19, 2017.

HCAHPS Survey. hcahpsonline.org. http://www.hcahpsonline.org/globalassets/hcahps/survey-instruments/mail/jan-1-2018-and-forward-discharges/click-here-to-view-or-download-the-updated-english-survey-materials.pdf. Published March, 2017. Accessed August 19, 2017.

Medicare.gov. Hospital value-based purchasing. https://www.medicare.gov/hospitalcompare/Data/hospital-vbp.html. Accessed August 19, 2017.

Medicare.gov. Mental health care (partial hospitalization). https://www.medicare.gov/coverage/partial-hospitalization-mental-health-care.html. Accessed August 19, 2017.

Medicare.gov. Quick facts about payment for outpatient services for people with Medicare part B. https://www.medicare.gov/Pubs/pdf/02118.pdf. Updated March 2015. Accessed August 19, 2017.

Medicare.gov. Survey of patients' experiences (HCAHPS). https://www.medicare.gov/hospitalcompare/Data/Overview.html. Accessed August 19, 2017.

QualityNet. Fiscal year 2017 measures hospital value-based purchasing. http://www.qualitynet.org/dcs/ContentServer?c=Page&pagename=QnetPublic%2FPage%2FQnetTier3&cid=1228775522697. Accessed August 19, 2017.

QualityNet. Hospital inpatient quality reporting (IQR) program overview. https://www.qualitynet.org/dcs/ContentServer?c=Page&pagename=QnetPublic%2FPage%2FQnetTier2&cid=1138115987129. Accessed August 19, 2017.

QualityNet. Measures hospital-acquired condition (HAC) reduction program. https://www.qualitynet.org/dcs/ContentServer?c=Page&pagename=QnetPublic%2FPage%2FQnetTier3&cid=1228774294977. Accessed August 19, 2017.

QualityNet. Overview hospital-acquired condition (HAC) reduction program. https://www.qualitynet.org/dcs/ContentServer?c=Page&pagename=QnetPublic%2FPage%2FQnetTier2&cid=1228774189166. Accessed August 19, 2017.

QualityNet. Scoring hospital value-based purchasing (HVBP). http://www.qualitynet.org/dcs/ContentServer?c=Page&pagename=QnetPublic%2FPage%2FQnetTier3&cid=1228772237147. Accessed August 19, 2017.

Reinhardt U. The pricing of U.S. hospital services: chaos behind a veil of secrecy. *Health Aff*. 2006;25(1):57-69. http://content.healthaffairs.org/content/25/1/57.full. Accessed July 6, 2017.

Sutton JP, Washington RE, Fingar KR, Elixhauser A. Characteristics of safety-net hospitals, 2014. Agency for Healthcare Research and Quality. https://www.ncbi.nlm.nih.gov/books/NBK401306/. Published October 25, 2016. Accessed August 19, 2017.

5

Advanced Practitioners to the Rescue
How Other Providers Are Paid

Christopher A. Clyne, MD, MBA
Britton Jewell, DO, MHA

Health care organizations would not be able to function as well as they do without advanced level practitioners. As the U.S. population is aging, advanced level practitioners are being called upon to fill the increased need for health care providers. They will need to practice at the top of their fields and will likely require greater autonomy. This chapter focuses on the roles of these advanced practitioners, how the major payers pay them, and the impact they have on our health care system.

HISTORY

In the 1960s, the need for primary care physicians grew because of increases in urban populations and lack of access to physicians in rural areas. In response to this shortage, advanced practitioner roles, including nurse practitioners (NPs) and physician assistants (PAs), were created.

In 1965, a physician named Henry Silver and a nurse named Loretta Ford created the first NP program at the University of Colorado. This program focused on expanding the traditional role of nurses to include more advanced additional clinical duties, such as history taking and physical examinations. The initial emphasis was placed on pediatric patients, but quickly expanded to all ages and many specialties. NP programs grew across the United States modeled after this first program.

The origins of PAs began in 1965 when physician Eugene Stead created the first PA program at Duke University. This training program was modeled after the military medical corps and focused on training advanced practitioners in 2 years. The first students were from the military medical corps themselves. These new practitioners were termed physician assistants (PAs) because they worked under a licensed physician to assist in many clinical roles, including complex surgeries. This program served as the model for expansion across the United States.

CHANGING ROLES REQUIRE CHANGING TERMINOLOGY: ADVANCED PRACTICE PROFESSIONALS DO NOT DELIVER "MID-LEVEL" HEALTH CARE

An advanced practice professional (APP) refers to a clinical provider who has undergone specialized education, training, certification, and licensure that allows her/him to provide many health care–related services with varying degrees of independence and with different levels of specialization. They are not physicians but may perform certain procedures and prescribe some medications.

The education and training of these professionals was developed originally with the goal of providing assistance to, and extending the services of, primary care physicians. The greatest need seemed to be in underserved areas. APPs now practice in every state, in many specialties, and in all settings. They can prescribe medications, including controlled substances, in all 50 states and Washington, D.C.

The term "mid-level practitioner" was established by the US Department of Justice's Drug Enforcement Administration (DEA) to identify a group of individual practitioners for the purpose of monitoring controlled substances. According to the DEA, Office of Diversion Control: Pursuant to Title 21, Code of Federal Regulations, Section 1300.01(b28):

> "the term mid-level practitioner means an individual practitioner, other than a physician, dentist, veterinarian, or podiatrist, who is licensed, registered, or otherwise permitted by the United States or the jurisdiction in which he/she practices, to dispense a controlled substance in the course of professional practice. Examples of mid-level practitioners include, but are not limited to, health care providers such as nurse practitioners, nurse midwives, nurse anesthetists, clinical nurse specialists and physician assistants who are authorized to dispense controlled substances by the state in which they practice."[1]

Medicare uses the term "nonphysician practitioner" to describe advanced practice nurses and PAs. The term "mid-level" connotes a level of the care that is not of the highest caliber and has, therefore, become replaced by the more appropriate term "advanced practice professional or advanced practice provider" (APP).

WHAT ADVANCED PRACTICE PROFESSIONALS DO AND HOW THEY ARE PAID

The Versatile Nurse Practitioner

As of 2017, there were over 230,000 licensed NPs in the United States—almost 90% of NPs were trained in programs focused on primary care. The role of the NP has evolved from that of a low-level assistant to one with advanced privileges and responsibilities. They can prescribe medications, including controlled substances, in all 50 states and Washington, D.C. As of 2017, NPs have full practice rights in 22 states and D.C., reduced practice rights in 16 states, and restricted practice rights in 12 states.

Full practice means that the state allows NPs to evaluate, treat, diagnose, and prescribe medications for patients independent of physician oversight. *Reduced practice* means that the state has limited at least one area of NP practice and requires collaboration with a physician. *Restricted practice* means that the state has limited at least one area of NP practice and requires physician oversight. Figure 5-1 shows a map of these practice rights that vary by state regulation and licensure laws.

It is important to be familiar with the different state laws in your area of practice.

The Mighty Physician Assistant

At the end of 2016, there were over 115,000 certified PAs in the United States. All states require collaboration with a physician; however, the specifics of the scope of practice can vary widely from state to state and can be determined by the supervising physician, allowing a broad range of practice for the PA.

Like NPs, PAs can evaluate, treat, diagnose, and prescribe medications for patients. However, unlike NPs, a physician must supervise all PAs. As of 2017, PAs can prescribe medications in all states, but prescribing of controlled substances is limited in eight states. Thirty-six states allow the scope of practice to be determined on an individual basis between the PA and supervising physician. In all, 30 states allow flexibility with direct supervision requirements and 28 states allow flexibility with cosignature requirements. Only 11 states allow physicians to supervise an unlimited number of PAs. Most states place limits, such as two or four.

REIMBURSEMENT METHODS

The APPs considered in this section are advanced practice registered nurses (APRNs), PAs, and anesthesiologist assistants (AAs). The different types of APRNs are listed as follows:

- NPs
- Certified registered nurse anesthetists (CRNAs)
- Certified nurse midwives (CNMs)
- Clinical nurse specialists (CNSs)

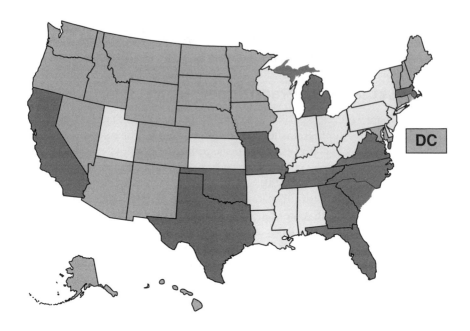

■ **Full Practice**
State practice and licensure laws provide for nurse practitioners to evaluate patients, diagnose, order and interpret diagnostic tests, initiate and manage treatments—including prescribe medications—under the exclusive licensure authority of the state board of nursing. This is the model recommended by the Institute of Medicine and National Council of State Boards of Nursing.

□ **Reduced Practice**
State practice and licensure law reduce the ability of nurse practitioners to engage in atleast one element of NP practice. State requires regulated collaborative agreement with an outside health discipline in order for the NP to provide patient care or limits the setting or scope of one or more elements of NP practice.

■ **Restricted Practice**
State practice and licensure law restricts the ability of a nurse practitioners to engage in atleast one element of NP practice. State requires supervision, delegation or team-management by an outside health discipline in order for the NP to provide patient care.

Figure 5-1 2017 nurse practitioner state practice environment. American Association of Nurse Practitioners. 2017 nurse practitioner state practice environment. https://www.aanp.org/images/documents/state-leg-reg/stateregulatorymap.pdf. Updated February, 2017.

Medicare Reimbursement

APPs usually bill under the physicians they work with when they are supervised. On these occasions, the physician is reimbursed at 100% of the Medicare contracted rate.

When APPs bill independently, they are reimbursed at 85% of the Medicare contracted rate (except for nurse anesthetists and nurse midwives who are reimbursed at different rates of the fee schedule).

The passage of the Balanced Budget Act of 1997 by Congress allowed Medicare to reimburse APPs independently if they are in a facility (hospital or other health care facility) or practicing "incident to" a physician in an office setting.

The *incident to* provision refers to services provided by APPs (PA, NP, CNM, and CNS) when the supervising physician is:

- Personally involved in the initial service
- Continues to participate in the patient's care
- Physically available (in the office area) during the encounter

One example of this provision would be if an APP sees an established patient in the office for a chronic problem without new problems. As long as a physician is "available" during the encounter and the patient was seen initially for the same problem by the MD/DO, the APP may bill and be reimbursed at 100% of the physician fee schedule.

CRNAs and AAs are reimbursed at a rate of 80% of the anesthesia fee schedule. CNMs are reimbursed at a rate of 100% of the physician fee schedule.

PAs, NPs, CRNAs, and CNSs are also subject to the Medicare Access and CHIP Reauthorization Act of 2015, which established the Merit-Based Incentive Payment System and Advanced Alternative Payment Models (see Chapter 1).

Medicaid Reimbursement

Medicaid reimburses services according to the specific state managed care program (eg, health maintenance organization) or as a fee-for-service agreement. Because each state program may vary, APP services may be reimbursed at an equal or lesser rate than physicians.

Private Insurance Reimbursement

Private insurers set their own reimbursement rates, which may (or may not) be similar to Medicare rates. Some insurers may bill services under the supervising physician or under the mid-level practitioner. It is necessary to check each insurers policy for reimbursement to advanced practitioners.

PRESENT AND FUTURE IMPACT ON HEALTH CARE DELIVERY

Since 1997, advanced level providers have grown greatly in numbers and have expanded their territories and scope of practice. The Bureau of Labor Statistics projects 38% growth in the number of PAs and 31% growth in the number of NPs, CNMs, and CRNAs for 2012 to 2022.

It is estimated that by 2020, the shortage of primary care physicians in the United States will exceed 20,000. The main force driving this increased need is the growth of a population that is living longer than ever before. The Affordable Care

Act (Obamacare) that became law in 2010 and provides health coverage for an additional 20 million (+) Americans through the Medicaid expansion is another contributor to the growing deficit in primary care providers. The future impact of the Affordable Care Act is uncertain in these politically charged times.

As the gap in primary care access widens, the cost of health care in the United States is also growing and now exceeds 17% of gross national product—the highest in the world. One solution to this dilemma has been to increase numbers and expand the roles of these advanced practitioners. NPs and PAs have been shown to be effective physician extenders and substitutes that improve the quality of care without increasing cost.

Deployment of these additional advanced practitioners could reduce the projected shortage of primary care providers to less than 6500 by 2020, thus expanding necessary health care access to remote and underserved regions, softening the physician shortage, and helping to reduce the cost of health care.

The numbers and roles of APPs continue to evolve with growing health care needs and changing legislation. They have been important providers of health care services to local hospitals and practices, as well as to underserved and rural areas. One certainty in the world of uncertain health care policy is that these APPs will become even more important in our health care future.

Reference

1. Drug Enforcement Administration. Mid-level practitioners authorization by state. http://www.deadiversion.usdoj.gov/drugreg/practioners/index.html. Accessed September 24, 2017.

Recommended Resources

American Academy of PAs. PA Scope of Practice. https://www.aapa.org/wp-content/uploads/2017/01/Issue-brief_Scope-of-Practice_0117-1.pdf. Updated January 2017. Accessed September 24, 2017.

American Academy of PAs. Third-party reimbursement for PAs. https://www.aapa.org/wp-content/uploads/2017/02/3rd_Party_Reimbursement_2017_FINAL.pdf. Updated January 2017. Accessed September 24, 2017.

American Association of Nurse Practitioners. Fact sheet: Medicare reimbursement. https://www.aanp.org/practice/reimbursement/68-articles/325-medicare-reimbursement. Published 2013. Accessed September 24, 2017.

American Association of Nurse Practitioners. Nurse practitioners. https://www.aanp.org/images/about-nps/npgraphic.pdf. Published June 2017. Accessed September 24, 2017.

American Association of Nurse Practitioners. 2017 nurse practitioner state practice environment. https://www.aanp.org/images/documents/state-leg-reg/stateregulatorymap.pdf. Updated February 2017. Accessed September 24, 2017.

Barton Associates. PA scope of practice laws. https://www.bartonassociates.com/locum-tenens-resources/pa-scope-of-practice-laws/. Updated April 28, 2017. Accessed September 24, 2017.

Bishop CS. Advanced practitioners are not mid-level providers. *J Adv Pract Oncol.* 2012;3(5):287-288. https://www.ncbi.nlm.nih.gov/pmc/articles/PMC4093350/. Published September 1, 2012. Accessed September 24, 2017.

Bureau of Labor Statistics. Nurse Anesthetists, Nurse Midwives, and Nurse Practitioners. https://www.bls.gov/ooh/healthcare/nurse-anesthetists-nurse-midwives-and-nurse-practitioners.htm. Published December 17, 2015. Accessed September 24, 2017.

Centers for Medicare & Medicaid Services. Advanced practice registered nurses, anesthesiologist assistants, and physician assistants. https://www.cms.gov/Outreach-and-Education/Medicare-Learning-Network-MLN/MLNProducts/Downloads/Medicare-Information-for-APRNs-AAs-PAs-Booklet-ICN-901623.pdf. Published October 2016. Accessed September 24, 2017.

Centers for Medicare & Medicaid Services. "Incident to" services. https://www.cms.gov/Outreach-and-Education/Medicare-Learning-Network-MLN/MLNMattersArticles/downloads/se0441.pdf. Updated August 23, 2016. Accessed September 24, 2017.

Comparison: Medicare's "Incident-To" vs. "Split / Shared" visits. UC San Diego Health Sciences. https://healthsciences.ucsd.edu/compliance/resources/Documents/2015_09%20Comparison%20Medicare%20Incident.pdf. Updated September 13, 2015. Accessed September 24, 2017.

Eilrich FC. The economic effect of a physician assistant or nurse practitioner in rural America. *JAAPA*. 2016;29(10):44-48. http://journals.lww.com/jaapa/Fulltext/2016/10000/The_economic_effect_of_a_physician_assistant_or.8.aspx. Accessed September 24, 2017.

Health Resources & Services Administration. Projecting the Supply and Demand for Primary Care Practitioners Through 2020. https://bhw.hrsa.gov/health-workforce-analysis/primary-care-2020. Published November 2013. Updated October 2016. Accessed September 24, 2017.

Huang L. Cost-effectiveness of nurse practitioners. Social Impact Research Experience. http://repository.upenn.edu/sire/37. Published July 25, 2016. Accessed September 24, 2017.

Kaiser Family Foundation. Medicaid benefits: nurse practitioner services. http://www.kff.org/medicaid/state-indicator/nurse-practitioner-services/?currentTimeframe=0&sortModel=%7B%22colId%22:%22Location%22,%22sort%22:%22asc%22%7D. Accessed September 24, 2017.

Kohler S. The development of the nurse practitioner and physician assistant professions. Center for Strategic Philanthropy & Civil Society. https://cspcs.sanford.duke.edu/sites/default/files/descriptive/nurse_practitioners_and_physician_assistants.pdf. Accessed September 24, 2017.

Morgan PA, Shah ND, Kaufman JS, Albanese MA. Impact of physician assistant care on office visit resource use in the United States. *Health Serv Res.* 2008;43(5 pt 2):1906-1922. doi:10.1111/j.1475-6773.2008.00874.x. Published July 28, 2008. Accessed September 24, 2017.

Morris J. Optimizing the value of advanced practice providers. Studer Group. https://www.studergroup.com/resources/articles-and-industry-updates/insights/august-2016/optimizing-the-value-of-advanced-practice-provider. Published August 12, 2016. Accessed September 24, 2017.

National Commission on Certification of Physician Assistants. 2016 statistical profile of certified physician assistants. http://www.nccpa.net/Uploads/docs/2016StatisticalProfileofCertifiedPhysicianAssistants.pdf. Published March, 2017. Accessed September 24, 2017.

Westgate A. Advanced practitioners: expanded role, bigger impact. Managed Healthcare Executive. http://managedhealthcareexecutive.modernmedicine.com/managed-healthcare-executive/news/advanced-practitioners-expanded-role-bigger-impact. Published September 11, 2015. Accessed September 24, 2017.

6

If It Ain't Written It Ain't Done
Basics of Documentation and Electronic Health Records

Christopher A. Clyne, MD, MBA
Britton Jewell, DO, MHA

"Observe, record, tabulate, communicate."

—Sir William Osler (1849-1919)

HISTORY

Medical record-keeping dates back at least to the ancient Greeks who kept logs of patient's cases and remedies for certain ailments. The purpose of those rudimentary records did not differ from the purpose of medical documentation today—to record and communicate the patient's history and the findings, thoughts, questions, and actions of the practitioner to other practitioners who may be involved in the patient's care.

The records of practitioners (until recently) have been hand-written and reflected the personalities of the author. There were no standards. Notes could be concise or wandering, clear or searching, readable or undecipherable.

Dr. Lawrence Weed introduced standardization of clinical documentation in the 1960s as an attempt to avoid medical errors, reduce redundancies in tests and procedures, promote clarity and purpose in the treatment of patients, and provide unambiguous and concise communication to other practitioners. His 1968 seminal article on the subject of clinical documentation, "Medical Records that Guide and Teach" is the foundation of modern clinical documentation and familiar to all medical students and medical-professionals who have been through a basic history and physical (H&P) course.

The medical record has become the repository for patients' health information, a vessel for education, a reservoir for data and research, a legal document more reliable than a physician's (or patient's) memory, and the evidence of a practitioner's work product for which they are paid.

The coincident explosion of technology and research in the late 20th century resulted in a meteoric rise in medical diagnoses, treatments, and a shift from "anecdotal" medicine to "evidence-based" medicine. The collection of data became a necessity for academics, researchers, practitioners, insurers, and the government. The use of forms and standardized approaches to medical conditions became ubiquitous in an attempt to collect, analyze, and communicate information efficiently. The possibility of treating populations of patients with common conditions (eg, diabetes, obesity, heart disease, and AIDS) to provide benefit to large numbers of patients at a low cost became a priority. All of this coincided with an explosion of technology, thus enabling the storage of massive amounts of data.

ELECTRONIC HEALTH RECORD

The electronic health record (EHR) was developed to organize and structure data in an effort to improve the quality of health care and reduce cost. "The primary goal of EHR-generated documentation should be concise, history-rich notes that reflect the information gathered and are used to develop an impression, a diagnostic and/or treatment plan, and recommended follow-up."[1]

The codification of medical information provided a means of memorializing the thought processes and actions of practitioners, recording doctor–patient interactions (for medical and legal purposes), building a reservoir of data for education and research, and providing a platform for the payers (insurers, employers, patients, and government) to judge work product and establish a formula for remuneration.

PURPOSES OF CLINICAL DOCUMENTATION

Patient Care, Communication, and Education

The problem-oriented medical record was designed to improve decision-making, treatment, and communication to other members of the patient's care team. An organized medical record can provide not just important documentation for these challenges but also a platform for quality improvement, education, population health initiatives, and research.

Risk Management

The average physician spends an estimated 11% of an assumed 40-year career (51 months) with an unresolved, open malpractice claim.[2]

Malpractice cases involving no payment to the patient do not mean they are no cost to the doctor. The average claim takes 4 to 5 years to resolve. During that time, the physician is under threat of not only losing a case decided "by a jury of his or her peers" but may have "punitive damages" attached that are not covered by malpractice insurance and put personal properties and earnings at risk. The case is frequently deemed "news-worthy," and the physician and family may find themselves on the front page of the local newspaper. She or he must attend countless attorney meetings and depositions. The stress can be destructive to a practice and a family. Medical malpractice laws, which determine whether a doctor is negligent in treating (or failing to treat) a patient on the basis of the standard of care, vary from state to state, but across the land, courts have long established clinical documentation to be discoverable, and the existence of an unaltered contemporaneous medical record is considered to be a more trusted source of truth than the memory of a physician or patient. In legal terms, if it isn't written down, it didn't happen. See Chapter 10 for more information on malpractice and health law.

EHRs have made defensive documentation easier. The effort to provide as much data as possible, however, has led to a source of "note bloat," where some conclude that superfluous negative findings, irrelevant documentation, and differential diagnoses dilute and obscure important clinical findings and lead to a glossing over the record by a frequently bored reader, resulting in diluted and missed information.

Coding and Billing

Evaluation and Management

Medicare and Medicaid billing is based solely on physician documentation. Evaluation and Management (E/M) coding developed by the American Medical Association and the Centers for Medicare and Medicaid Services (CMS) is the process by which physician–patient encounters are translated into five-digit current procedural terminology (CPT) codes to facilitate billing. These are the numeric codes that are submitted to insurers for payment. Every billable procedure has its own individual CPT code.

The CPT codes that describe physician–patient encounters are often referred to as "E/M codes." There are different E/M codes for different types of encounters, such as office visits or hospital visits. Within each type of patient encounter, there are different levels of care. An office visit has five levels of care for this type of encounter. For example, the 99213 code is often called a "level 3" office visit because the code ends in a "3" and also because it is the third "level of care" for that type of visit. The codes range from the lowest—99211 to the highest—99215, which correlates to the first through fifth levels of care, respectively. Each patient care encounter may be viewed as a unique procedure that requires specific documentation.

Before the release of the E/M guidelines in 1995 and 1997, physician billing for nonprocedural work was based on a self-assessment and self-attestation. The level of cognitive investment and decision-making complexity and/or time spent was left to the professional judgment of the physician. Medical records were comprised of notes that were often difficult to read and to whose voracity and veritas were difficult to verify. The E/M guidelines were developed as a way to standardize, measure, and codify the cognitive component of patient care. The emphasis was no longer on what was reportedly done, rather on what was documented.

There are three *key components* to each encounter; each containing four sub-categories, each of which is composed of various rules, rubrics, and checklists that make E/M documentation extremely complicated and challenging. To optimize reimbursement and minimize litigation and penalties for "fraud" (billing without the proper documentation), hospitals and medical practices have developed entire departments with experts called "clinical documentation improvement (CDI)" specialists.

The Key Components of Evaluation and Management Documentation

The documentation for E/M services is based on three *key components*:

History

The history is designed to provide a narrative that provides information about the clinical problems being addressed in each encounter and is composed of four basic components:

- Chief complaint (CC)
- History of present illness (HPI)
- Review of systems (ROS)
- Past medical, family, and social histories (PFSH)

There are five "levels of history" that require different combinations of the components: from "problem focused,"—the lowest level—requiring only CC and HPI, to "comprehensive extended,"—the highest level—requiring all components of the "history." The "level of history" is composed of required CC and HPI for all levels. ROS and PFSH are included for detailed and comprehensive levels of history.

Physical Examination

There are four levels of intensity and documentation for the PE. There are differences between the 1995 and 1997 E/M guidelines for defining levels of the PE. The 1995 guidelines give the physician a wide margin to document the PE on the basis of body areas or systems. The 1997 guidelines are specific requiring documenting the examination using predefined landmarks or "bullets."

    a. Problem focused: one to five bullets from one or more organ systems
    b. Expanded problem focused: six bullets from any organ system
    c. Detailed examination: two or more bullets from six organ systems or 12 bullets from 2 or more organ systems
    d. Comprehensive: two bullets from each of nine organ systems

Medical Decision Making

Medical Decision Making (MDM) reflects the complexity of the collection, assimilation, and analysis of all of the information required to make medical decisions for the patient during the encounter. The official rules for interpreting the MDM are identical for both the 1995 and 1997 E/M guidelines.

    There are four levels of MDM of incrementally increasing complexity:

    a. Straightforward
    b. Low complexity
    c. Moderate complexity
    d. High complexity

    MDM levels of complexity are determined by tabulating the number and types of clinical problems addressed, the number and types of data used and reviewed for the encounter, and the level of risk to the patient (Figure 6-1). The level of risk

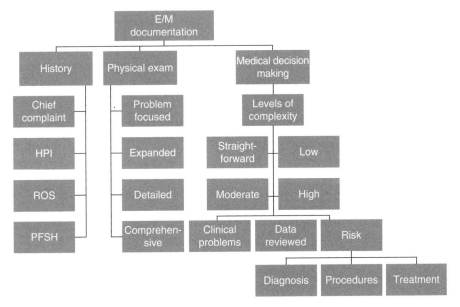

Figure 6-1 Example of a rubric for determining level of medical decision making showing the three key areas of E/M documentation with their associated components. E/M, evaluation and management; HPI, history of present illness; PFSH, past medical, family, and social histories; ROS, review of systems.

is determined by the type of presenting illness (eg, acute myocardial infarction), the diagnostic procedures involved in the encounter (eg, cardiac catheterization), and the treatment options for the patients (eg, open-heart surgery).

It is highly recommended that each provider become very familiar with the CDI departments in their practices and institutions and take advantage of the many excellent webinars, tutorials, and courses offered in this important and ever-changing area of "medicine."

INPATIENT OR OUTPATIENT (OBSERVATION)?

Payments for Medicare patients differ depending on whether the patient is an inpatient (Medicare Part A—Inpatient Prospective Payment System) or outpatient/observation (OBS) (Medicare Part B—Outpatient Prospective Payment System). The "Two-Midnight Rule" was introduced in 2015 as an attempt to prospectively determine patient status with reliance on the physician/practitioner's judgment, while providing clear guidelines for payment status. Inpatient status may be financially more favorable for some patients, as they may be responsible for 20% of the bill not covered by Medicare Part B for OBS/outpatient services. Additionally, Medicare patients who require skilled nursing facilities must be inpatients for a minimum 3-day stay in order to cover the cost. Time spent in hospital as an OBS patient does not count toward the 3-day inpatient stay. Hospitals are paid a lump sum for bundled services, including emergency department, labs, pharmacy, bed costs, and so on for the OBS patient.

Practitioners are expected to determine whether a patient will require more than two midnights in the hospital to qualify for inpatient payment status. Clear documentation of the patient's illness (diagnosis), associated conditions (severity of illness), and expected evaluation and treatment (procedures and plan of action) are the determinants of whether Medicare will consider the patient to be an inpatient or an OBS patient. It is important to be familiar with the specific language that is accepted by CMS and other insurers to justify a specific condition/diagnosis (coded as a "Diagnosis Related Group" [DRG]), procedure, and hospital status because this determination directly impacts both the patient and the institution.

Patients who remain after two midnights must:

a. be discharged,
b. remain in OBS at the hospital's expense when the delay is because of a systemic delay and not a change in patient status,
c. change to inpatient status with clear documentation as to the reason for the change.

KNOW THE LANGUAGE

It is not enough to simply document the admitting, visit, and discharge problems with the associated challenges and action plan. There is a specific language replete with reimbursement buzzwords that you, as the *attending physician/responsible practitioner*, must become familiar with in order to receive reimbursement for an encounter. It is impossible to cite and list all possible diagnostic nomenclature here. Here are a few examples of *Dos and Don'ts* of documenting. Because this field is always changing, it is strongly advised to keep close to the CDI personnel in your office or institution for updates and tutelage.

Examples of Documentation Deficiencies and Optimization

Syncope

Generally admitted as OBS—unless it can be linked to a medical condition that justifies inpatient status:

- Syncope due to pulmonary embolus
- Syncope due to ventricular tachycardia
- Syncope due to severe sepsis

Heart Failure

No:

- Left ventricular dysfunction
- Diastolic dysfunction
- Congestive heart failure
- Exacerbation of heart failure

Yes: Be descriptive using *acuity, type, linkage to associated conditions, and onset*

- *Acuity:* acute, chronic, or acute on chronic systolic, diastolic, or systolic and diastolic (combined) heart failure (equals exacerbation)
- *Type:* systolic, diastolic, combined systolic and diastolic heart failure
  - (May use *heart failure with preserved/reduced ejection fraction* as substitute for systolic and diastolic heart failure—HFpEF/HFrEF)
- *Link to associated conditions:* acute combined systolic and diastolic heart failure due to ischemic cardiomyopathy/chronic hypertension/alcoholic cardiomyopathy
- *Onset*: include time of onset such as if present on admission

Urinary Tract Infections

Be as specific and inclusive as possible-include type, organism identification, associated conditions, organ involvement, time of onset.

- No: "Urinary tract infection (UTI)"
- Yes: "UTI with (systemic inflammatory response syndrome/sepsis/severe sepsis) due to (type of organism [bacteria]/identification of organism [*Escherichia coli*]) associated organ failure/conditions (complicated by acute kidney failure; due to indwelling Foley; causing hyperkalemia). Present on admission."

WHAT'S A "QUERY?"

Not all documentation is complete at the time of coding. Often, proper documentation is lacking and needs clarification. The clinical documentation specialist may communicate the apparent deficiency to the responsible practitioner in a "query."

The American Health Information Management Association describes a query as "a routine communication and education tool used to advocate complete and compliant documentation."[3]

The query is both an inquiry for clarification and a tool to provide the necessary documentation for the patient's encounter. It is crucial to patient care, risk management, as well as coding and billing. Queries may be communicated in several ways: flagged notices in the chart, secure e-mails, notices in the EHR, but all must be consistent with the medical record and not introduce new information and should never attempt to lead the practitioner to a particular diagnosis. The following are examples of typical queries found in the EHR that give the practitioner many choices, including free texting, to better clarify a diagnosis.

Please Clarify Etiology of Diagnosis

Syncope

- Cardiac arrhythmia (type)
- Cerebrovascular accident
- Orthostatic hypotension
- Anxiety
- Carotid sinus
- Hypoglycemia
- Other etiology
- Clinically unable to determine
- Disagree

Altered Mental Status

- Toxic metabolic encephalopathy
- Hepatic encephalopathy
- Wernicke encephalopathy
- Hypoxic encephalopathy
- Metabolic encephalopathy
- Dementia with delirium
- Other etiology
- Clinically unable to determine
- Disagree

CONCLUSION

"Successful clinical documentation improvement (CDI) programs facilitate the accurate representation of a patient's clinical status that translates into coded data. Coded data is then translated into quality reporting, physician report cards, reimbursement, public health data, and disease tracking and trending."[4]

As a practitioner, you must clearly document and justify your level of involvement for each patient encounter. Further, you must adhere to the current documentation guidelines in order to accurately preserve the medical record, manage risk, and optimize reimbursement for each type of involvement.[1] Clinical documentation and the coding systems (International Classification of Diseases 10th Revision) are living processes that are forever improving and changing. Partnering with your CDI specialist is critical to enabling the transfer of accurate information, avoiding malpractice and/or fraud accusations, and recouping just remuneration for your work.

You can be the most conscientious practitioner with the best of intentions, but *if ain't written, it ain't done!*

References

1. Kuhn T, Basch P, Barr M, Yackel T; Medical Informatics Committee of the American College of Physicians. Clinical documentation in the 21st century: executive summary of a policy position paper from the American College of Physicians. *Ann Intern Med.* 2015;162(4):301-303. http://annals.org/aim/article/2089368/clinical-documentation-21st-century-executive-summary-policy-position-paper-from. Accessed September 25, 2017.
2. Seabury SA, Chandra A, Lakdawalla DN, Jena AB. On average, physicians spend nearly 11 percent of their 40-year careers with an open, unresolved malpractice claim. *Health Aff (Millwood)*. 2013;32(1):111-119. http://content.healthaffairs.org/content/32/1/111.full.pdf+html. Accessed September 25, 2017.
3. Haugen MB, Tegen A, Warner D; American Health Information Management Association. Fundamentals of the legal health record and designated record set. *J AHIMA.* 2011;82(2):44-49. http://library.ahima.org/PB/DesignatedRecordSet#.Wcmhe8iGPIU. Accessed September 25, 2017.
4. American Health Information Management Association. Clinical documentation improvement. http://www.ahima.org/topics/cdi. Accessed September 25, 2017.

Recommended Resources

Centers for Medicare and Medicaid Services. Evaluation and management services. https://www.cms.gov/Outreach-and-Education/Medicare-Learning-Network-MLN/MLNProducts/Downloads/eval-mgmt-serv-guide-ICN006764.pdf. Published August 2017. Accessed September 25, 2017.

Centers for Medicare and Medicaid Services. Fact sheet: two-midnight rule. https://www.cms.gov/Newsroom/MediaReleaseDatabase/Fact-sheets/2015-Fact-sheets-items/2015-07-01-2.html. Published July 1, 2015. Accessed September 25, 2017.

E/M University. Introduction and definitions. http://emuniversity.com/Definitions.html. Accessed September 25, 2017.

Schwartz SK. Defensive medicine versus value-based care. *Med Econ.* 2016;93(6):17-18, 20-22. http://medicaleconomics.modernmedicine.com/medical-economics/news/defensive-medicine-versus-value-based-care. Accessed September 25, 2017.

Weed LL. Medical records that guide and teach. *N Engl J Med.* 1968;278:593-600. http://www.nejm.org/doi/full/10.1056/NEJM196803142781105. Accessed September 25, 2017.

7

Charging Responsibly
Clinical Documentation Integrity and Risk Adjustment

Christopher A. Clyne, MD, MBA
Britton Jewell, DO, MHA

INTRODUCTION

Because the U.S. health care system is progressively incentivizing the value of care that is provided, clinical documentation has become increasingly scrutinized and used for more than just documenting the patient's treatment plan. Documentation is now used for submitting insurance claims and determining reimbursements, among many other uses. Because of the importance of accurate, timely, and complete documentation, clinical documentation improvement (CDI) programs have emerged as a necessity for health care organizations to optimize their reimbursement strategies and improve the quality of care provided.

Let us briefly summarize what we have covered so far with regard to billing and coding. Chapter 1 discusses the basics of billing for Medicare for providers (current procedural terminology [CPT] codes) and hospitals (diagnosis-related group [DRG] and ambulatory payment classifications [APCs]). Chapter 3 describes in more detail how providers are paid, including pay-for-performance initiatives. Chapter 4 describes in more detail how hospitals are reimbursed and describes Medicare's quality programs. Chapter 6 describes the basics of clinical documentation, including the Evaluation and Management (E/M) system of coding and electronic health records (EHRs). This chapter explains why optimizing this documentation is not only important for high-quality patient care but also for appropriate billing and coding. It also discusses the evolving role of documentation to profile population risk and predict future reimbursement for millions of covered patient lives.

HISTORY OF CLINICAL DOCUMENTATION IMPROVEMENT

With the implementation of EHRs and need to analyze large volumes of data, clinician documentation has additionally become important for quality improvement and utilization management initiatives, as well as reimbursement optimization, risk adjustment, and risk management. As a result, the clinical documentation specialist (CDS) role was created in order to assist providers, health care organizations, and insurers in documentation management and improvement.

CDSs are usually registered nurses, but may also have a background in coding. They are primarily responsible for reviewing the clinical details of a patient's condition, diagnosis, and progress. They must ensure that all information pertaining to a patient is captured and written down to accurately describe the severity of illness and treatment plan. CDI programs were created to facilitate this process, with a focus on capturing the correct DRG and case mix index (CMI). The CMI is the average of the DRGs and corresponds to the severity of illness. DRGs that accurately reflect a higher severity of illness will equate to a higher CMI, longer length of stay, higher expected mortality, and, therefore, a higher reimbursement for a health care organization. CDI also protects an organization from audits and supports appropriate billing practices.

A CDS also functions to educate physicians and other providers about correct documentation practices. CDI is not traditionally a part of medical education, but is increasingly being recognized as being a component of high-quality patient care.

RISK ADJUSTMENT

On January 1, 2014, three Affordable Care Act (ACA) provisions went into effect that prevented insurance companies from charging higher premiums or denying coverage for preexisting conditions, and established the premium subsidies for health plans on the exchanges. In order to prevent insurance companies from "cherry-picking" the healthiest people to cover and avoiding enrolling sick people, the ACA provided three additional provisions: the "three Rs" of *risk adjustment, reinsurance,* and *risk corridors.* The reinsurance and risk corridor programs expired in 2016; however, the risk adjustment program is permanent. The reinsurance program paid health plans that enrolled sicker (and costlier) people, and the risk corridor program prevented health plans from losing or gaining too much money outside a set range. These programs attempted to stabilize premium costs by helping insurance plans cover the sickest people.

The risk adjustment program is a permanent provision of the ACA. This program was created to prevent insurers from picking only the lowest risk individuals to cover. It accomplishes this by having health plans with lower risk individuals pay into a fund that makes payments to health plans with higher risk individuals. This program incentivizes quality and value rather than saving money by only covering healthy people. All plans in the small group and individual insurance exchanges must participate. Prior to 2017, states could opt to oversee their own programs. However, as of 2017, the federal government runs the risk adjustment program in every state.

The insurance plans must give or receive money to each other based on the financial risk of their plan members. This risk is calculated for each enrollee based on an individual risk score, or risk adjustment factor (RAF). The individual risk score is made up of the enrollee's demographics (age and sex) and medical diagnoses. The medical diagnoses, expressed in *International Classification of Diseases, 10th Edition (ICD-10)* codes, are assigned to a hierarchical condition category (HCC).

HIERARCHICAL CONDITION CATEGORIES

The HCC model has been used by the Centers for Medicare and Medicaid Services (CMS) for Medicare Advantage plans since 2004 and is also used in Medicare Shared Savings Program Accountable Care Organizations (ACOs). For health plans offered on the insurance exchanges, CMS uses the Department of Health and Human Services (HHS) HCC model, an adapted form of the CMS-HCC model. The HCC model is a prospective system that seeks to predict future expenses for enrollees by reviewing the *ICD-10* data for every individual. It does not matter the setting in which the *ICD-10* code is documented in the patient's record (inpatient, outpatient). Not all *ICD-10* codes correspond to an HCC. For 2017, of the 69 000 *ICD-10* codes, only about 10 000 of them map to one of 79 HCCs. The HCCs are chronic diseases, such as cancer, diabetes, and chronic kidney disease, which are thought to contribute more to long-term health care costs. The HCCs are "hierarchical" because for one disease process, there may be multiple different HCCs to describe the severity. For example, if data submitted to CMS have *ICD-10* codes that are assigned to HHC 28 (Cirrhosis of Liver) and HHC 27 (End-Stage Liver Disease), only HCC 27 applies to risk adjustment because it is of a higher severity. However, not all HCCs are hierarchical because an individual can have more than one, such as HCC 108 (Vascular Disease) and HCC 134 (Dialysis Status). In addition, the model takes into account having multiple diseases simultaneously by adjusting for interactions between diseases.

The RAF score is calculated based on the individual's demographics and each HCC the individual is assigned. The demographics and HCCs are each given their own score, which are added together to equal the total RAF. Each year, CMS publishes a "denominator" to multiply the total RAF by to equal the dollar amount the enrollee is expected to cost.

Risk Scores Matter

For plans with capitated rates, such as Medicare Advantage plans, higher risk scores equal higher payments (per member per month). For ACOs, higher risk scores mean higher (easier) targets to achieve cost savings. For plans offered on the insurance exchanges, the total risk scores for all members are averaged and then adjusted for other factors, such as plan rating (platinum, gold, silver, bronze, and catastrophic), amount of cost sharing, and geographic area. The plans with lower risk scores have to pay into the system, and plans with higher risk scores receive money. In 2014, about $4.6 billion was transferred between health insurers. Additionally, many state Medicaid programs also use risk adjustment but utilize one of several different models (such as MedicaidRx, Diagnostic Cost Groups [DxCG], and others) that are outside the scope of this chapter.

If the risk scores are not calculated appropriately, cost savings will be harder to achieve, and the health care organization (or providers) may be less profitable, or even lose money. As we have already discussed, risk scores are calculated based on the *ICD-10* codes. This is why documentation is so important! A provider cannot change a patient's demographics, but they can document their medical conditions more accurately to appropriately capture the severity of the patient's illness. Risk scores are updated each year, so it is important to consistently capture each individual's diagnoses every year.

Remember, not all diagnoses (*ICD-10* codes) risk adjust!
Examples:

- I49.9 *Cardiac dysrhythmia, NOS* does not risk adjust, but I48.91 *Atrial fibrillation* does
- E66.9 *Obesity, NOS* does not risk adjust, but E66.01 *Morbid obesity* does
- J18.9 *Pneumonia, NOS* does not risk adjust, but J13 *Pneumonia due to Streptococcus pneumoniae* does

Table 7-1 presents a 76-year-old female patient, showing the change in the RAF when different diagnoses are coded. An "X" in the box indicates the disease process was not coded. When documented appropriately in the medical record and then coded, the RAF shows in the appropriate box. Notice how the RAF increases significantly as the amount of HCCs increases.

For 2017, the denominator is $9 185.29. Therefore, multiplying the RAF by the denominator equals an estimated cost for this enrollee of $5 446.88, $6 530.74, and $16 625.37, respectively, based on the chronic conditions that are coded. That is a greater than $10 000 difference for just this one individual. Now you can understand how risk adjustment accounts for billions of dollars in potential loss/revenue for health insurers and why it is important for providers to document appropriately.

TABLE 7-1   Risk Adjustment Coding Example

No Conditions Coded		Some Conditions Coded		All Chronic Conditions Coded	
76-y-old female	0.442	76-y-old female	0.442	76-y-old female	0.442
Medicaid eligible	0.151	Medicaid eligible	0.151	Medicaid eligible	0.151
DM with complications	X	DM without complications	0.118	DM with complications	0.368
Vascular disease	X	Vascular disease	X	Vascular disease	0.299
CHF	X	CHF	X	CHF	0.368
Disease interaction (DM + CHF)	X	Disease interaction (DM + CHF)	X	Disease interaction (DM + CHF)	0.182
Total RAF	**0.593**	**Total RAF**	**0.711**	**Total RAF**	**1.810**

Abbreviations: CHF, congestive heart failure; DM, diabetes mellitus; RAF, risk adjustment factor.
From Hawaii Medical Service Association. HMSA success in 2017—risk adjustment, quality measures, and care of older adults. https://hmsa.com/portal/provider/HMSA_Success_In_2017_Quality_Changes_Risk_Adjustment_Care_for_Older_Adults_011117.pdf. Published January 10, 2017. Accessed April 9, 2018.

Revenue Integrity

Risk adjustment brings up an important topic of revenue integrity. With the shift away from fee-for-service, reimbursements depend more on the value of care that is provided. Higher value means higher quality and lower costs. Provider documentation provides written evidence of the quality of care that is provided.

Revenue integrity refers to the methods that health care organizations and providers use to receive accurate reimbursements. This encompasses many different aspects such as clinical documentation integrity (CDI), coding, billing, pricing of services, and complying with governmental and private insurer's policies, regulations, and requirements. Not complying with any of these processes can mean decreased revenue that an organization is otherwise entitled to. Health care providers play a role in revenue integrity through their accurate documentation that captures the patient's severity of illness and treatment plan.

ETHICS OF CODING

With risk adjustment becoming a larger part of determining reimbursements, it has become even more important to ensure that documentation and coding is performed based on sound ethical principles. The Government Accountability Office estimated that in 2016, about $16 billion in inappropriate payments were paid out to Medicare Advantage plans mostly because of inaccurate coding. In 2017, the US Justice Department filed a suit against UnitedHealth Group Inc (*U.S. ex rel.*

Poehling v. UnitedHealth Group Inc et al, U.S. District Court, Central District of California, No. 16-cv-08697) that claims that UnitedHealth overbilled Medicare by over $1 billion by submitting inaccurate diagnoses for their Medicare Advantage enrollees. At the time of this publication, this case has yet to have been decided.

The American Health Information Management Association publishes a set of standards for ethical coding, that cover such concepts as:

- Being accurate, consistent, and complete to ensure quality data.
- Following all requirements and data set definitions.
- Using only the codes and data that are supported by health record documentation.
- Consulting as needed with providers to clarify or obtain additional documentation before assigning final codes.
- Practicing coding with integrity.
- Advancing coding knowledge through continuing education.
- Maintaining confidentiality at all times.
- Refusing to participate in or address any activity intended to misrepresent data or conceal unethical coding.[1]

ACCURATE DOCUMENTATION

Many CDSs recommend providers to utilize the acronym "MEAT" to appropriately document with HCC in mind. MEAT stands for:

- "Monitor—signs, symptoms, disease progression, disease regression
- Evaluate—test results, medication effectiveness, response to treatment
- Assess/Address—ordering tests, discussion, review records, counseling
- Treat—medications, therapies, other modalities"[2]

This is in addition to the E/M system of documentation discussed in Chapter 6. The MEAT system should be applied to every diagnosis to support the associated HCC code and insulate against audits. Some additional strategies for HCC documentation include:

- The HCC codes should be captured at least once every calendar year.
- The *ICD-10* codes should be appropriately documented in the medical record.
- Causality or linking diagnoses should be described (eg, peripheral neuropathy secondary to type II diabetes mellitus).
- All documentation/reports from specialty referrals, imaging, and diagnostic testing should be reviewed (including the body of the report, not just the impression).

CONCLUSION

CDI encompasses every aspect of a patient's encounter with the health care system. Every time a patient interacts with a health care organization or provider, a record is kept of the encounter. CDI departments and CDSs are important resources that help ensure revenue integrity and quality standards are upheld by scrutinizing documentation practices. The financial benefits of appropriate risk adjustment are tangible; however, this only exists to improve the quality and value of care that health care providers are delivering to their patients.

These organizations must have appropriate funding if they are to continue to provide a high standard of care. The integrity and financial impact of clinical documentation will ultimately rely on the provider's understanding of how clinical documentation affects reimbursement and population health, and a commitment to provide comprehensive and honest documentation.

References

1. American Health Information Management Association House of Delegates. American Health Information Management Association standards of ethical coding [2016 version]. http://bok.ahima.org/CodingStandards#.WrRO9ejwbIU. Published December 2016. Accessed April 9, 2018.
2. Cassano HJ. HCCs: easy as 1, 2, 3 (the culture of MEAT). *JustCoding News: Outpatient*. March 19, 2014. http://www.hcpro.com/content.cfm?content_id=302031. Accessed April 9, 2018.

Recommended Resources

Cassano C. The rewarding role of clinical documentation specialist. *American Nurse Today*. October 2014. https://www.americannursetoday.com/rewarding-role-clinical-documentation-specialist/. Accessed April 9, 2018.

Centers for Medicare and Medicaid Services. Announcement of calendar year (CY) 2017 medicare advantage capitation rates and medicare advantage and part D payment policies and final call letter. https://www.cms.gov/Medicare/Health-Plans/MedicareAdvtgSpecRateStats/Downloads/Announcement2017.pdf. Published April 4, 2016. Accessed April 9, 2018.

Cox C, Semanskee A, Claxton G, Levitt L. Explaining health care reform: risk adjustment, reinsurance, and risk corridors. Washington, DC: Kaiser Family Foundation. https://www.kff.org/health-reform/issue-brief/explaining-health-care-reform-risk-adjustment-reinsurance-and-risk-corridors/. Published August 17, 2016. Accessed April 9, 2018.

Empire BlueCross. CMS-HCC risk adjustment model (V22). https://www11.empireblue.com/provider/noapplication/f2/s2/t4/pw_g312847.pdf?refer=ehpprovider. Updated February 2018. Accessed April 9, 2018.

Hawaii Medical Service Association. HMSA success in 2017—risk adjustment, quality measures, and care of older adults. https://hmsa.com/portal/provider/HMSA_Success_In_2017_Quality_Changes_Risk_Adjustment_Care_for_Older_Adults_011117.pdf. Published January 10, 2017. Accessed April 9, 2018.

Hawaii Medical Service Association. Risk adjustment and clinical documentation. https://hmsa.com/portal/provider/Risk_Adjustment_and_Clinical_Documentation_SLIDES_032917.pdf. Published March 28, 2017. Accessed April 9, 2018.

Health Care Compliance Association. Clinical documentation improvement (CDI) programs: what role should compliance play? https://www.hcca-info.org/Portals/0/PDFs/Resources/Conference_Handouts/Regional_Conference/2016/orange-county/HatzelBeltonprint3.pdf. Published June 17, 2016. Accessed April 9, 2018.

Lagassse J. Physician practices examine risk adjustment coding in wake of federal lawsuits. *Healthcare Finance News.* September 25, 2017. http://www.healthcarefinancenews.com/news/physician-practices-examine-risk-adjustment-coding-wake-federal-lawsuits. Accessed April 9, 2018.

Natale C. Why clinical documentation improvement is so important to hospitals. *Healthcare IT News.* April 4, 2012. http://www.healthcareitnews.com/blog/why-clinical-documentation-improvement-so-important-hospitals. Accessed April 9, 2018.

Raymond N. U.S. can sue UnitedHealth in $1 billion Medicare case, judge rules. *Reuters.* February 13, 2018. https://www.reuters.com/article/us-unitedhealth-lawsuit/u-s-can-sue-unitedhealth-in-1-billion-medicare-case-judge-rules-idUSKCN1FX25S. Accessed April 9, 2018.

Schoen M, Najera M. Achieving revenue integrity in hospitals and health systems. *Healthc Financ Manag.* 2012;66(9):114-120.

Yeatts JP, Sangvai DG. HCC coding, risk adjustment, and physician income: what you need to know. *Fam Pract Manag.* 2016;23(5):24-27. https://www.aafp.org/fpm/2016/0900/p24.html. Accessed April 9, 2018.

8

Big Brother Is Watching
Quality and Compliance

Christopher A. Clyne, MD, MBA
Britton Jewell, DO, MHA

INTRODUCTION

It could be said that health care in the United States is going through a quality movement. "Quality" and "value-based" are terms you are likely hearing with increasing frequency throughout the industry. Quality improvement objectives are becoming a part of everyday work flows and are becoming a part of the culture of many organizations, from hospitals and clinics, to health systems and health plans. Providing high-quality care is not only important for patient interactions but also becoming a necessity to maintain compliance with organizational rules, goals, and values. This chapter helps the reader to better understand what is meant by "quality," why it is necessary, where it came from, and how quality is achieved and maintained in modern health care.

HISTORY OF THE QUALITY MOVEMENT

Attempts to improve the quality of care provided is not a new phenomenon, but it wasn't until the observations of the Hungarian obstetrician, Ignaz Semmelweis, in the mid-1800s, who noted that nurse midwives at Vienna General Hospital had an infection rate one-third that of doctors. He attributed this disparity to the practice of handwashing by the midwives and noted a similar reduction in purpuric fever and mortality when he employed handwashing before deliveries. His practice was ignored until Pasteur's germ theory was accepted and Joseph Lister also showed the life-saving impact of practicing operative hygiene.

The modern quality movement was spawned from the realization that health care outcomes were improved when the stakeholders collaborated to establish standardized definitions and goals; systems for health care delivery; evidence-based practices; methods for monitoring, reviewing, incentivizing good, and reprimanding poor performance; quality improvement tools; transparency and public reporting; and medical education practices designed to incorporate evolving medical and health-related knowledge.

There have been numerous quality models and agencies developed over the decades to improve quality and safety that have resulted in changes in infrastructure and practices and have exposed some of the deficiencies of current practices. None of these have been as influential in redefining the goals and methods of quality improvement as the Institute of Medicine's (IOM's) 1999 publication *To Err Is Human: Building a Safer Health Care System* and a follow-up report in 2001 *Crossing the Quality Chasm: A New Health System for the 21st Century.* These two reports generated shockwaves throughout the industry and pointed a spotlight on the large amount of life-threatening medical errors in our health care system that were occurring with increasing frequency and without public knowledge. These critical reports led to the development of the National Quality Forum (NQF) whose goal it was to "define national goals and priorities for health care quality improvement, and to build national consensus around these goals and to endorse standardized performance metrics for quantifying and reporting on national healthcare quality efforts."[1]

The NQF established and defined the "gold standard" for health care performance measures used by many agencies (including Centers for Medicare and Medicaid Services [CMS]) for accreditation and reimbursement.

The IOM defines *quality* as "the degree to which health services for individuals and populations increase the likelihood of desired health outcomes and are consistent with current professional knowledge."[2]

Quality as measured by patient outcomes and adherence to practice and performance standards has become a key requirement for accreditation of hospitals, clinics, health care agencies, and individual practitioners. It has also become an important variable in the reimbursement calculus with incentives and penalties to institutions and individuals based on quality performance measures.

QUALITY OF CARE IN THE UNITED STATES

Why Is It Important to Measure Health Care Quality?

As my father used to say, "You got your health, then you got everything."

Nothing is as important to most people from every country and culture as good health. People have a desire to be healthy and understand that we as providers of care must have benchmarks and standards of health in order to treat patients toward health. An individual's health often requires data to be analyzed and measured against standards. For example, we recognize the normal range of sodium in the blood for men and women. An "abnormal" electrocardiogram means something to the patient and to the practitioner. Conclusions about health require standards, and standards require data.

It is important to keep the population healthy. Our individual health depends, in part, on our neighbors' health. Think of the "Black Plague" or the yellow fever infectious endemics of old. More currently, immunization practices have reduced morbidity and mortality from contagious diseases such as polio, measles, and influenza.

Population health is also important to keep our economy moving and growing. It is critical to a thriving economy to have a healthy workforce, but health care is expensive. In 2016, national health expenditures hit $3.35 trillion, almost 18% of gross domestic product, and about $10 345 for every man, woman, and child. We must be able to determine what is worth paying for and how much to pay. This is called *value.*

American health care is shifting from fee-for-service to value-based health care where reimbursement is aligned with performance and outcomes. The CMS is spearheading efforts to improve quality and efficiency while reducing cost through programs such as the Medicare Access and CHIP Reauthorization Act (MACRA) of 2015, the Merit-based Incentive Program (MIPS), and Advanced Alternative Payment Models (APM), which will base reimbursement to hospitals and providers on performance, patient outcomes, and patient satisfaction. These new mandated programs will consolidate and replace previous quality initiatives, including Medicare Meaningful Use, the Value-based Payment Modifier, and the Physician Quality Reporting System (PQRS).

How Is Quality Measured?

Quality measurement implies outcomes data. Various agencies collect data in numerous ways with different goals. Data may be collected from claims data sheets, public data (eg, death certificates and census data), disease registries, prospective funded studies, and patient surveys. These data may be used, for example, to compare the health of populations in various regions or nations, disease states, treatment outcomes, population trends, or the efficiencies (cost and value-based outcomes) of entire health systems.

The Organization for Economic Co-operation and Development (OECD) is an organization of 35 countries whose mission is to stimulate economic growth and trade. They collect and compare mortality and key health systems data across member countries.

In 2015, the IOM published *Vital Signs: Core Metrics for Health and Health Care Progress.* This group of committee experts was able to condense and standardize from thousands of measures of individual health and of health systems— some 15 core measures that serve as benchmarks for optimal health outcomes at a lower cost for Americans.

For a view of current *U.S. Population Health Measures, U.S. Quality of Care Measures,* and *International Comparisons of Population Health and Quality Measures,* please refer to the following links from the Peterson–Kaiser Health System Tracker:

- Appendix: Measuring the quality of healthcare in the United States. http://www.healthsystemtracker.org/wp-content/uploads/2015/09/Appendix-Measuring-the-quality-of-healthcare-in-the-U.S1.pdf. Published September 10, 2015.
- How has the quality of the US healthcare system changed over time? https://www.healthsystemtracker.org/chart-collection/quality-us-healthcare-system-changed-time/. Published September 9, 2015.

Who Is Watching?

What follows is a partial list of agencies involved in the field of health care quality monitoring and assessment.

Federal Government

- Department of Health and Human Services (HHS): www.hhs.gov
  - Administration for Children and Families: www.acf.hhs.gov
  - Administration for Community Living: www.acl.gov
  - Agency for Healthcare Research and Quality: www.ahrq.gov
    - National Quality Strategy: www.ahrq.gov/workingforquality/index.html
  - Agency for Toxic Substances and Disease Registry: www.atsdr.cdc.gov
  - Assistant Secretary for Administration: www.hhs.gov/about/agencies/asa/index.html
  - Assistant Secretary for Financial Resources: www.hhs.gov/asfr
  - Assistant Secretary for Health: www.hhs.gov/ash
  - Assistant Secretary for Legislation: www.hhs.gov/about/agencies/asl/index.html
  - Assistant Secretary for Planning and Evaluation: aspe.hhs.gov
  - Assistant Secretary for Preparedness and Response: www.phe.gov/preparedness/Pages/default.aspx
  - Assistant Secretary for Public Affairs: www.hhs.gov/aspa
  - Center for Faith-Based and Neighborhood Partnerships: www.hhs.gov/partnerships
  - Centers for Disease Control and Prevention: www.cdc.gov
  - CMS: www.cms.gov
    - Medicare: www.medicare.gov
    - Medicaid: www.medicaid.gov
    - Hospital Value-Based Purchasing Program
    - Hospital Readmissions Reduction Program
    - Hospital-Acquired Condition Reduction Program

- ◆ Hospital Inpatient Quality Reporting Program
- ◆ Meaningful Use Program
- ◆ Physician Value-Based Modifier Program
- ◆ PQRS
- Departmental Appeals Board: www.hhs.gov/about/agencies/dab/index.html
- Food and Drug Administration (FDA): www.fda.gov
  - ◆ MedWatch: www.fda.gov/Safety/MedWatch/default.htm
- Health Resources and Services Administration: www.hrsa.gov/index.html
- Immediate Office of the Secretary: www.hhs.gov/about/agencies/staff-divisions/immediate-office-secretary/index.html
- Indian Health Service: www.ihs.gov
- National Institutes of Health: www.nih.gov
- Office for Civil Rights: www.hhs.gov/ocr/index.html
- Office of Global Affairs: www.hhs.gov/about/agencies/oga/index.html
- Office of Inspector General (OIG): oig.hhs.gov
- Office of Intergovernmental and External Affairs: www.hhs.gov/iea/index.html
- Office of Medicare Hearings and Appeals: www.hhs.gov/about/agencies/omha/index.html
- Office of the Chief Technology Officer: www.hhs.gov/about/agencies/cto/index.html
- Office of the General Counsel: www.hhs.gov/about/agencies/ogc/index.html
- Office of the National Coordinator for Health Information Technology: www.healthit.gov
- Substance Abuse and Mental Health Services Administration: www.samhsa.gov

State and Local Governments

- Departments of Health
- Child and Adult Protective Services
- State Medical Boards (see Appendix 1)
- State Medical Associations

Nongovernmental Agencies

- National Committee for Quality Assurance: www.ncqa.org
- The Joint Commission: www.jointcommission.org
- OECD: www.oecd.org
- IOM: iom.nationalacademies.org
- Institute for Healthcare Improvement: www.ihi.org

- Leapfrog Group: www.leapfroggroup.org
- NQF: www.qualityforum.org
- Patient-Centered Outcomes Research Institute: www.pcori.org

Some Tools for Quality Improvement

- Healthcare Effectiveness Data and Information Set
- Comparative Effectiveness Research
- Lean
- Six Sigma
- Peer Review
- Board Exams
- Evidence-Based Guidelines and Standards of Practice
- Credentialing Processes
- Electronic Health Records (EHRs): Pharmacy Prompts, Resources, Reporting
- Hospital Accreditation Based on Quality and Safety Measures: The Joint Commission
- Licensing Review Processes
- Checklists Preceding Procedures and Processes
- Healthcare Leadership Training and Empowerment Programs
- Reporting Mechanisms and Agencies
- Risk Adjustment Analysis

As you can see, there are multiple stakeholders who have an interest in health care quality. Each of these organizations or entities may create rules, laws, regulations, or guidelines (some voluntary or involuntary) to ensure that health care organizations provide high-quality care. The practice of upholding these rules and laws is termed *compliance.*

WHAT IS COMPLIANCE?

Compliance bridges the gap between laws/regulations/rules/guidelines, financial responsibilities, legal responsibilities, risk management, ethics, organizational culture, and arguably the ultimate success of a business. Compliance in the health care industry can refer to many different issues:

- Patient privacy protection (Health Insurance Portability and Accountability Act [HIPAA])
- Ethical billing and coding
- Following federal and state laws and guidelines
- Appropriate training of employees and practitioners
- Creating plans for reporting and correcting breaches
- Complying with audits
- Avoiding fraud and abuse

HISTORY OF COMPLIANCE IN HEALTH CARE

Compliance issues in public health are mostly governed by federal and state agencies. In 1906, the FDA was created to improve safety and oversight. In 1973, the Drug Enforcement Administration was created, spurring organizations to form their own compliance programs to ensure they were following the laws, rules, and regulations required in their industry. In 1996, the HIPAA was passed, which fundamentally changed the health care industry.

THE HEALTH INSURANCE PORTABILITY AND ACCOUNTABILITY ACT

In 1996, the HIPAA was created to address several broad issues:

- Guide the use of EHRs
- Manage heath care data
- Protect patient privacy
- Secure patient health data
- Guide the portability of medical data
- Allow individuals to keep their health insurance when leaving their job

This section will not provide a comprehensive overview of HIPAA but will address the most important issues related to compliance.

The US Department of Health and Human Services (HHS) was responsible for creating the HIPAA "Rules," which became health industry standards. These rules focused on protecting the privacy and security of protected health information (PHI).

The HIPAA Privacy Rule establishes the privacy of PHI, which includes any information that can individually identify someone, such as demographics, social security number, medical record number, and photograph. This rule requires health care organizations to provide a Notice of Privacy Practices to patients. In 2009, as part of the American Recovery and Reinvestment Act, the Health Information Technology for Economic and Clinical Health Act was passed, which modified HIPAA's privacy and security rules. It endorses the use and standardization of EHRs, requires organizations to notify patients if a security breach occurs, and notifies HHS and the media if over 500 people are affected.

The HIPAA Security Rule establishes the protection of PHI and specifically addresses electronic data. It requires administrative, physical, and technical safeguards to be established. Administrative safeguards include appointing a chief security officer, employee and staff training, controlling access to data, and recognizing and reporting security breaches. Physical safeguards include ensuring the physical safety of servers and databases, backing up data, and controlling the viewing of data. Technical safeguards include creating usernames and passwords, encryption, and automatic logoffs.

FEDERAL LAWS GOVERNING COMPLIANCE

False Claims Act

The False Claims Act was passed all the way back in 1863 and prevents the intentional submission of false or fraudulent payment claims. This includes Medicare payments thatare subject to fraud and abuse.

Anti-kickback Statute

In 1972, the Anti-kickback Statute was passed, making it a felony to intentionally offer, pay, solicit, or receive compensation for a referral, or to cause reimbursable services to be created under a federal health care program. This includes patient referrals or any other reimbursable item or service under a federal health care program.

Stark Law

The Stark Law was passed in 1989 and prohibits particular financial relationships between a referring physician and any individual/organization that bills Medicare or Medicaid. A physician cannot refer to that individual/organization if themselves or any immediate family members have a financial relationship (there are exceptions to the application of this law).

MAINTAINING COMPLIANCE

HIPAA requires every organization to have a compliance officer to make sure all requirements are followed. Organizations must install appropriate security safeguards to ensure that patient information is protected. In addition, employees and staff must undergo compliance training. There must be procedures in place for a patient to file a complaint. They may contact the Office of Civil Rights or the HIPAA Program Office. Organizations may face civil or criminal penalties for violations. Civil penalties consist of fines, whereas criminal penalties include fines and possible prison time of up to 10 years for the most egregious violations.

The OIG from the HHS provides guidance for health care institutions/providers to evaluate their compliance programs. There are multiple areas to evaluate:

- Access
- Accountability
- Review/approval process
- Quality
- Assessment
- Code of conduct
- Updates

- Understanding
- Compliance plan
- Confidentiality statements
- Enforcement
- Board of director involvement
- Compliance budget
- Compliance committees

- Compliance officer
- Staffing
- Culture
- Incentives
- Performance evaluations
- Risk assessments
- Involvement of legal counsel
- Conflict of interest
- Employee disclosure and screening
- Exit interviews
- High-risk screening
- Licensure
- Vendor screening and oversight
- Training
- Awareness
- Communication
- Competency
- Volunteers
- Reporting system
- Monitoring and auditing work plans

- Corrective action plans
- Auditors
- Nonretaliation
- Consistency
- Documentation
- Promotion criteria
- Guidelines for conducting an investigation
- Quality and consistency of investigations
- Communication of investigation outcomes
- Training, professionalism, independence, and competency of investigators
- Timeliness of response
- Remedial measures
- Root cause analysis
- Government inquiries/ investigations
- Monitoring result

As you can see, compliance programs involve basically every aspect of the organization. Health care organizations conduct internal and external audits to ensure their compliance programs are functioning as intended.

CONCLUSION

Quality and compliance are important to all stakeholders of the health care industry. Patients benefit from receiving better care from practitioners who have access to their data while respecting their privacy. Practitioners benefit from utilizing better patient data to make diagnostic and treatment decisions. Payers benefit from receiving accurate and timely claims data. The health care industry as a whole will continue to improve care quality to benefit the entire population.

References

1. American Pharmacists Association. Quality measures—quality organizations. https://www.pharmacist.com/quality-measures-quality-organizations. Accessed April 20, 2018.
2. Institute of Medicine (US) Committee on Quality of Health Care in America. *Crossing the Quality Chasm: A New Health System for the 21st Century.* Washington, DC: National Academies Press; 2001. https://www.ncbi.nlm.nih.gov/books/NBK222274/. Accessed April 20, 2018.

Recommended Resources

AAPC.com. HIPAA. https://www.aapc.com/healthcare-compliance/hipaa.aspx. Accessed April 20, 2018.

AAPC.com. What is healthcare compliance? https://www.aapc.com/healthcare-compliance/healthcare-compliance.aspx. Accessed April 20, 2018.

Appendix: Measuring the quality of healthcare in the U.S. Peterson-Kaiser health system tracker. http://www.healthsystemtracker.org/wp-content/uploads/2015/09/Appendix-Measuring-the-quality-of-healthcare-in-the-U.S1.pdf. Published September 10, 2015. Accessed April 20, 2018.

Department of Health and Human Services, Office of Inspector General. Measuring compliance program effectiveness: a resource guide. https://oig.hhs.gov/compliance/101/files/HCCA-OIG-Resource-Guide.pdf. Published March 27, 2017. Accessed April 20, 2018.

Institute of Medicine (US) Committee on Core Metrics for Better Health at Lower Cost. In: Blumenthal D, Malphrus E, McGinnis JM, eds. *Vital Signs: Core Metrics for Health and Health Care Progress.* Washington, DC: National Academies Press; 2015. https://www.nap.edu/read/19402/chapter/1. Accessed April 20, 2018.

Institute of Medicine (US) Committee on Quality of Health Care in America. In: Kohn LT, Corrigan JM, Donalson MS, eds. *To Err is Human: Building a Safer Health System.* Washington, DC: National Academies Press; 2000. https://www.ncbi.nlm.nih.gov/books/NBK225182/. Accessed April 20, 2018.

Kamal R, Cox C. How has the quality of the US healthcare system changed over time? Peterson-Kaiser Health System Tracker. https://www.healthsystemtracker.org/chart-collection/quality-us-healthcare-system-changed-time/. Published September 9, 2015. Accessed April 20, 2018.

MacKessy J. Knowledge of good and evil: a brief history of compliance. *The Finance Professionals' Post.* http://post.nyssa.org/nyssa-news/2010/05/a-brief-history-of-compliance.html. Published May 26, 2010. Accessed April 20, 2018.

Marjoua Y, Bozic KJ. Brief history of quality movement in US healthcare. *Curr Rev Musculoskelet Med.* 2012;5(4):265-273. doi:10.1007/s12178-012-9137-8.

National Quality Forum. NQF's Mission and Vision. http://www.qualityforum.org/About_NQF/Mission_and_Vision.aspx. Accessed April 20, 2018.

Office of Corporate Compliance, The University of Chicago Medical Center. HIPAA Background. http://hipaa.bsd.uchicago.edu/background.html. Published October 23, 2006. Updated February 2010. Accessed April 20, 2018.

Organisation for Economic Cooperation and Development. OECD Health Statistics. https://www.oecd-ilibrary.org/social-issues-migration-health/data/oecd-health-statistics_health-data-en. Accessed April 20, 2018.

Record Nations. The history of HIPAA and the consequences of a HIPAA violation. https://www.recordnations.com/articles/history-hipaa/. Accessed April 20, 2018.

9

Your Virtual Presence
Navigating Social Media

Christopher A. Clyne, MD, MBA
Britton Jewell, DO, MHA

Social media has many advantages, such as helping to build your practice, assisting in finding a job, expanding your professional network, and maintaining relationships. There are many sites to choose from and some could have the unintentional effect of blurring the lines between your personal and professional lives. This chapter discusses which social media websites are the most useful for the health care professional and provides some helpful information to keep in mind when building your online presence.

USING SOCIAL MEDIA RESPONSIBLY

We shouldn't have to remind you that anything you post online is there forever, even if you delete it. It is good practice to keep your personal and professional social media profiles separate and to never post any patient information online, ever! It is tempting to rant about a rough day at work, but it is our recommendation to never post anything that could violate privacy laws even if the names or locations are changed. It is not worth the consequences, no matter if the chances of facing them are extremely low. A good rule of thumb is "If you wouldn't say it publicly, then don't write it down." With that being said, let's discuss the most popular social media websites.[1]

TOP SOCIAL MEDIA WEBSITES

Facebook: www.facebook.com

Almost everybody has a Facebook account for personal use. Using this site for professional purposes, as well as for your personal use, would blur that line between your personal and professional lives that we mentioned earlier. To avoid patient-friend requests, you could create a separate personal and professional account or create a professional page for your practice. You may wish to make your personal account private. This site can be a great networking tool for physician offices and getting your name out there.

LinkedIn: www.linkedin.com

This site is very similar to Facebook, but is only used for professional purposes. Your profile is basically an online resume or curriculum vitae. This site is great for professional networking, searching for job opportunities, and expanding your professional knowledge through reading insightful posts and articles.

Twitter: www.twitter.com

This is an extremely popular social media site that allows you to make posts limited to 140 characters or less. This is another site that you may wish to separate your personal and professional accounts. This is also a great site to read news posts and articles and can also be used to promote your practice.

Doximity: www.doximity.com

This site is very similar to LinkedIn, but is specifically focused on the health care field. Members must be physicians or other health care providers. This site is for networking and job searching. It would not be the best site to promote your practice because it is not open to the general public.

Blog Style Websites: www.blogger.com, www.wordpress.com

Many physicians have their own blogs to post about their own experiences or discuss various health topics. The two most popular free blog sites are Blogger and WordPress. These sites can be a great way to promote your practice, discuss your perspectives on health care, and connect with your audience.

QuantiaMD: www.quantiamd.com

This is a site exclusively for physicians and provides networking, continuing medical education activities, and learning opportunities. The more you interact with the site, the more "Q-Points" you can earn, which can be redeemed for Amazon.com gift cards.

Sermo: www.sermo.com

This is a social networking site only for physicians and is open to members from many different countries. There are over 800 000 members who go through a verification process and can remain anonymous. This site allows patient care collaboration as well as discussion on general topics.

Mayo Clinic Social Media Network: socialmedia.mayoclinic.org

This social network was created by the Mayo Clinic and is open to all health care providers, students, patients, and caregivers. There is a free basic membership that includes access to three free webinars per year, a blog, and a monthly e-newsletter. There are also premium memberships available for individuals or organizations that include access to 10 webinars per year, a weekly e-newsletter, conference discounts, and a discussion board.

WeMedUp: www.wemedup.com

This site is open to all health care professionals, administrators, and students. This site allows collaboration with research, case studies, and group discussion. It has information on employment opportunities, ability to create or participate in polls, and has discounts on medical supplies.

Student Doctor Network: www.studentdoctor.net

This is a very popular forum for medical and premedical students. Joining this site and contributing to the community by answering questions and providing advice is a good way to give back. It is always well appreciated and welcomed by the members.

HEALTH CARE PROVIDER RATING SITES

Your online presence can also be affected by forces outside your control, such as provider rating websites. These sites elicit feedback from patients where they can grade your services. There are many different sites that offer these services. Some of the most popular are listed in Table 9-1.

In addition, some of the most popular general rating sites such as Yelp (www.yelp.com) and Google Maps (maps.google.com) offer ratings for health care professionals as well.

Of these rating sites, there is not one that has emerged as the most popular. Word of mouth is still the best method to build your practice. It would take a lot

TABLE 9-1   Health Care Provider Rating Websites

www.healthgrades.com

www.ratemds.com

www.vitals.com

of time and energy to monitor all the rating websites out there. The best method to protect your online reputation is with a good bedside manner and with helpful and friendly office staff.

CONCLUSION

Social media can be an excellent tool to promote yourself and your practice. You must closely monitor the lines between personal and professional subject matter because you may not want certain information shared with your current or prospective patients. Your social media content can also affect your future job prospects, even if posted on your personal page. We recommend keeping your personal and professional accounts separate, but closely monitor what is posted on each. Your online reputation is affected by what you choose to say to others and by what others say about you, and rating websites provides an outlet to do so.

Reference

1. ReminderCall.com. 10 best social media sites for healthcare providers. https://www .remindercall.com/social-media-sites-for-healthcare-providers. Published July 7, 2016. Accessed July 10, 2017.

10

Protect Yourself
Medical Malpractice and Health Law

Christopher A. Clyne, MD, MBA
Britton Jewell, DO, MHA

With any luck, and a lot of effort, none of you reading this chapter will have experienced the dreaded medical malpractice lawsuit. We wish that we could be optimistic and write that as long as you adhere to good practices and never make a mistake that you are free from the roils and entanglements of the legal profession.

The truth is "that by the age of 65 years, 75% of physicians in low-risk specialties had faced a malpractice claim, as compared with 99% of physicians in high-risk specialties."[1]

The average medical malpractice lawsuit takes years to resolve and requires many hours of preparation away from your practice and family with attorneys in depositions and court, and countless hours of lost sleep and consternation. When a patient or family sues, the emotional wound takes a toll on the practitioner undermining confidence and trust in him- or herself, in the practitioner–patient relationship and, frequently, in the system that provides the platform for the suit.

Although most physicians recognize that there are episodes of negligence and malpractice—and that patients should be provided a means of protection and just compensation for errors or malpractice—they often respond that the system is not entirely fair.

The practitioner may wake up to find their name on the front page of the local newspaper as the physician/nurse/physician assistant named in a "negligence" suit, leading to feelings of humiliation, helplessness, and fear even before they have had a chance to defend themselves.

The actual legal process may also cause great resentment and anxiety. Although less than 5% of all cases will reach a courtroom settlement, the fear that a complicated medical case may be judged by a lay "jury of your peers" can be quite frightening, especially when the practitioner learns that the punitive damages that the Plaintiff's attorney may ask the judge to add to the complaint are **not covered by your medical malpractice insurance**, and a losing verdict could result in complete financial collapse for the defendant and family.

Being involved in a lawsuit can be extremely unpleasant, time consuming, lead to depression, disrupt family life and marriages, and impact the practitioner's ability and approach to practice in the future. Physicians contend that the threat of malpractice lawsuits forces them to practice defensive medicine, which, in turn, raises the cost of health care.

The purpose of this chapter is to inform you so that you are aware of some of the pitfalls that can lead to a lawsuit, and to provide suggestions to help you avoid a medical malpractice lawsuit. This chapter should be for educational purposes only. Please note that we are not providing or attempting to provide any legal advice. If you are involved with any lawsuit, medical malpractice or otherwise, we recommend to seek the advice of a qualified lawyer.

TORTS

A *tort* is "an act or omission that gives rise to injury or harm to another and amounts to a civil wrong for which courts impose liability."[2]

It is important to note that torts are a civil wrongdoing, not criminal; however, some torts can result in criminal liability, such as battery.

Types of Torts

Torts are divided into three types:

- *Negligent torts:* An unintentional act that results in harm
- *Intentional torts:* A deliberate act that results in harm
- *Strict liability torts:* Typically applies to product manufacturers and does not take intent into account

Negligence

Negligence is an unintentional act, or omission, that does not perform at least to the standard of a reasonable person under similar circumstances. It requires proof of four parts:

- Duty
- Breach of duty
- Injury
- Causality

In health care, clinicians have a *duty* to care for their patients. A *breach of duty* can occur when the standard of care is deviated from. The patient must experience harm, or an *injury*. The *cause* of the injury must be because of the breach of duty. In order to qualify for negligence, all of these criteria must be met. Negligence can result in malpractice, but not all cases of malpractice are because of negligence.

Intentional Torts

Intentional torts must be performed on purpose. Some common intentional torts that apply to the health care field are listed here, followed by a short definition or example.

- *Assault:* Intending to cause harm to the patient, or the patient believes harm may result.
- *Battery:* Touching a patient without their consent.
- *False imprisonment:* Holding a patient against their will. Avoiding this tort allows competent patients to leave the hospital against medical advice. Physical restraints are not necessary for this type of tort.
- *Emotional distress:* Patient suffering severe emotional distress.
- *Defamation:* Injury to reputation caused by defamatory statements, either spoken (*slander*) or written (*libel*).
- *Invasion of privacy:* Failure to uphold the confidential physician–patient relationship.
- *Wrongful death:* A patient death caused by wrongful acts.
- *Fraud:* Lying that results in financial gain, such as falsifying billing or insurance claims.

TORT REFORM

You may have heard the term "tort reform" when referring to medical malpractice cases. Tort reform, in the context of health care, refers to reforming the current malpractice system, usually limiting the amount of damages that can be rewarded to a patient or that a physician can pay. Many states have imposed their own tort reform laws, including limiting the dollar amount of damages.

Tort reform is a very politically charged issue. Proponents argue that tort reform will help to lower the practice of "defensive medicine" that will help to drive down health care costs. Opponents argue that tort reform will not allow injured patients to receive the amount of justice, in the form of monetary compensation, that they deserve. At the time of this publication, the Trump Administration has not been successful in passing any tort reform.

MEDICAL MALPRACTICE

Medical malpractice occurs when a health care provider deviates from the recognized "standard of care" in the treatment of a patient. The *standard of care* is defined as what a reasonably prudent medical provider would or would not have done under the same or similar circumstances. A malpractice claim exists if a provider's negligence causes injury or damages to a patient. The medical malpractice claim does not necessarily arise from "negligence."

Experiencing a bad outcome isn't always proof of medical negligence. An undesirable (bad) outcome for a patient, or a contentious relationship with a difficult family member or patient, may result in you being sued. Involvement in the care of a patient who sues the institution or another physician may also result in you being named in the suit. Although you cannot control every aspect of care or outcome for a patient, you can limit your risk.

Risk Management

"Risk management is a series of strategies designed to reduce the likelihood of injury to the patient, and when injury occurs, to reduce the likelihood that a suit results."[3]

Risks abound in the daily practice of medicine, from alleged diagnostic errors and inadequate follow-up, to errors in documentation and communication. The following are the top causes of malpractice suits. By recognizing what poses the greatest risk, physicians can create and implement formal policies and procedures to protect their practices and themselves.

Major Causes of Malpractice Suits

The top factors caused patient injury, based on review of the data, are:

- Alleged errors in clinical judgment (38%)
- Problems with technical skills (23%)
- Problems with communication (22%)
- Patient behaviors (20%)
- System failures (14%)
- Documentation deficits or errors (13%)

Medical Malpractice Payouts 2016

1. Dollars in payouts: $3.84 billion
2. Total payouts for medical malpractice: 12 142 (1 every 43 minutes)
3. Payouts resulting from judgments: 4%
4. Payouts resulting from settlements: 96%
5. Number 1 payout allegation: failure to diagnose

How to Protect Yourself From Medical Malpractice Lawsuits

AVOID

I think that we all would agree that it is in the best interest of every practitioner to AVOID a claim by a patient. Here are some suggestions for how to reduce risk:

Practice Evidence-Based Medicine

The #1 cause for a malpractice suit (mentioned earlier) is an error in judgment. As health care providers for each unique individual that we encounter, we must apply our *clinical judgment* for each patient and each case. This is actually what we get paid to do! Although we can't be perfect 100% of the time, we can provide excellent care and reduce risk by practicing **evidence-based medicine**. This requires that the practitioner is familiar with and employs the standard of care for each patient-related challenge and uses current resources when she or he is unfamiliar with an issue or treatment. Further, this requires keeping up to date with continuing medical education (CME) credits and following current guidelines and clearly documenting when and why you have chosen to deviate from those guidelines. These guidelines represent the medical profession's best judgment about when the scientific evidence backs a treatment or procedure. You can access the guidelines through the Department of Health and Human Services' National Guidelines Clearinghouse at https://www.ahrq.gov/research/findings/factsheets/errors-safety/ngc/national-guideline-clearinghouse.html.

Avoid Technical Errors—Easier Said Than Done

Everyone makes mistakes—but mistakes can be minimized if you follow a few basic principles:

Informed Consent

Informed consent is one of the most important elements of the patient–practitioner relationship. We may think of "informed consent" as applying only to the documents that a patient signs before a procedure. It is more than that. Each time we meet with a patient, we are asking their consent to ask the most personal questions and uncover secrets of habit and health. The process requires respectful engagement and communication if it is to be done correctly. When asking for consent to perform a test or procedure, we must use the same principles and take the time to clearly explain the risks and benefits, expected outcomes, the why's, and the alternatives for each patient. It is important that consent for a procedure should be obtained by the operator and not a surrogate. This might give the impression that the operator does not consider the procedure or the patient to be important enough for his or her time and lead to resentment should there be a problem. It is thus fitting that the patient expects to speak directly to the operator.

Informed consent is about managing a patient's/family's expectations. To do this, the practitioner must provide the proper information for the patient to make an informed and reasonable decision free of bias or coercion. By exchanging information, the patient not only becomes informed but becomes a partner in the decision-making process sharing responsibility with the medical team. The informed consent process protects both patients and practitioners.

Make a List

In any technical procedure—operation, chemotherapy delivery, and dental procedure—there are many steps each of which can derail a perfect outcome if left undone or done improperly.

Dr Atul Gawande recognized that "We miss stuff. We are inconsistent and unreliable because of the complexity of care." Inspired by the success of the airline industry in avoiding errors by using checklists, he studied the similar approach applied to technical/surgical procedures in medicine. His book *The Checklist Manifesto: How to Get Things Right* explains how the power of being organized and adhering to protocols and checklists can avoid errors in the operating room.

Adhere to standardized protocols where they exist for technical procedures and follow the same protocol each time. If one doesn't exist, create one with the assistance of the team of professionals involved in the procedure. Listen to the patient and to all members of the team. Pay attention to detail and to deviations. These suggestions may save a life and will certainly help to avoid errors.

Communicate Effectively

"'The issue that affects everything else [in malpractice litigation] is when patients are angry,' says Robin Diamond, RN, JD, senior vice president for patient safety and risk management for The Doctors Company. 'There might be some competency issues, but in the vast majority of cases when we go in we find an issue with the relationship between the patient and the physician.'"[4]

Each patient–practitioner relationship is unique and will require communication skills from all of the staff to develop a relationship of mutual respect, trust, and comfort. Encourage staff to bring the patient into the process as a respected partner—to communicate with them from the time they enter the office, hospital, or clinic to the time they leave. The front desk or admitting hospital staff person is the face of your practice. Provide training for your staff in telephone etiquette, professional demeanor, and techniques to deal with angry or dissatisfied patients.

If you and staff are welcoming and make patients who are waiting to see a practitioner, or for an operation/procedure feel looked after and not forgotten, patients are less likely to be angry and avoid the practice . . . or worse!

When you meet with a patient, take time to listen. Repeat what the patient has conveyed to you back to them so they know you were actively listening. Ask them questions and encourage their questions. Ask them to repeat their understanding of the information back to you. Close the loop at each encounter.

If you have limited time, tell them so they don't feel slighted if you are called out of the visit. When using a computer to enter data into the electronic health record (EHR), face the patient and take time to look at them and respond openly to questions. Repeat patient statements for clarity.

When explaining a diagnosis, treatment, or prognosis to a patient and family, use medically correct terms but avoid medical jargon. Use lay terms when possible. Use an interpreter when necessary. Identify the risks. Explain the short- and long-term outcome possibilities. Talk about alternatives. Let the patient enter into the decision-making process.

Follow-up is an important part of validating the partnership between practitioner and patient. Calling the patient with test results or to check up on them after a procedure closes the loop and helps to promote trust and loyalty. It is also important to follow up with referrals to other practitioners/specialists or testing locations for your patients. Have a process for checking that patients are properly scheduled; that the specialist is aware and has all pertinent records; and that the patient is aware of the appointment. This can be delegated to a staff member. Document that this was done and communicated to the patient.

Be Forthright

If you or your team made a mistake, disclose it. Moreover, you should be the one to inform the patient as soon as you realize that there was error/mistake/negligence. It looks (and is) bad when the patient learns that you knew of a medical error and said nothing. This erodes trust and results in an adversarial relationship between patient and provider. Explain the error in lay terms. Be clear and accept responsibility. Be honest. Apologize. Do not "throw someone else under the bus." This shows an unwillingness to accept responsibility and cowardice. Most patients and families understand that no provider or system is perfect. Further, if you are sued, it is far better to be on the record as an honest practitioner than one who is thought to hide from the truth.

It is important to inform and work together with the Risk Management team of your health care facility or practice when you identify a problem that suggests negligence or malpractice. They will provide good council on the best approach for disclosure, communication, avoidance of conflict (with the patient or family), and mitigation/remedy of harm or injury.

"Robin Diamond, RN, JD, senior vice president for patient safety and risk management for The Doctors Company, offers the following recommendations for enhancing patient satisfaction and reducing the likelihood of being sued:

For Physicians

- Acknowledge your limited time with the patient by saying, 'We only have a few minutes. Let's make the best use of it and get right to the issue.'
- When using an electronic health record, face the patient. Explain to the patient that this system will improve care and follow-up.
- If you sense that a patient is feeling hurried, explain to the patient how much time you have and then make sure that a staff member is available to answer as many questions as possible. Make sure the patient doesn't leave angry.
- Provide training for your staff in telephone etiquette, professional demeanor, and techniques to deal with angry or dissatisfied patients.
- Provide a safe, healthy environment for staff.

For Staff Members

- Immediately acknowledge the patient, even if you're on the phone.
- As soon as possible, greet the patient and confirm the time of the appointment. Immediately address any other issues, such as whether the physician is running late.
- If the patient is waiting in the reception area or treatment room, regularly check in with him or her to see if there is anything you can do, in addition to giving updates on how late the appointment may be.
- Ask if you can bring in a magazine, water, or other comfort items.

- When the patient is leaving the office, review any follow-up instructions and confirm that the patient understands—for example, ask the patient to repeat back when to return for the follow-up appointment.

Everyone Who Interacts with Patients

- Patients want to be heard.
- Patients want to be treated with respect.
- Patients want to ask questions and to have them answered.
- Patients want to know how to voice a concern or complaint and get a quick response."[4]

Document Everything!

The EHR has provided a way to document almost everything that takes place in a patient's care history. This has been both boom and bust for the practitioner. While these systems allow archiving and retrieval of large amounts of data that can be transferred among sites, assist in decision-making by providing reference resources/guidelines/checklists, deliver safety alerts to avoid errors, and encourage patients to access and participate in their own care, they also have drawbacks: they have a relatively steep learning curve and require a fair amount of training to use effectively. Productivity in the early stages of use is reduced by around 20%. Attention to inputting data by the practitioner during an encounter may result in creating a distance between patient and provider. Other types of errors can occur, including wrong clicks, missed information in a sea of data, and so on.

The EHR can be responsible for reducing or enhancing risk for the practitioner. If the information exists in the EHR, the practitioner is responsible for knowing it! That includes current and old medical encounters, diagnoses, meds, conditions, and so on. Everything that is entered or accessed is time coded and dated, and you own it!

Many systems are set up to provide alerts, such as drug allergies, incompatibilities, best practices, guidelines, and Black Box warnings. Do not disregard these. Read them carefully—you are responsible for their message.

Reconciling medications at the time of admission and discharge is standard practice for most practitioners. Every time you sign on to a patient's EHR, you are expected to review the current medications. Daily medication review used to be very time consuming and incomplete. The EHR has reduced medication errors and the burden of daily medication review and reconciliation.

There is a temptation with many versions of EHR to "cut and paste" repetitive information from a prior note into a current note. This may lead to inaccurate or irrelevant information if not updated on a daily basis. Further, the ease of incorporating preexisting data (labs, meds, and tests) and text into every note may lead to "note bloat," where the note is excessive in length filled with irrelevant information that dilutes important current clinical information. This may result in a failure to notice a change in status or an important test result. This also discourages the important transfer of current information in a narrative form where the practitioner can express his or her current analysis, impression, assessment, and plan on a daily

Table 10-1   Types of Malpractice Claims Related to the Electronic Health Records (EHR): System Factors Versus User Factors 2007 to 2014

EHR System Factors (eg, technology, design, security)	EHR User Factors (eg, user errors)
Failure of system design (10%)	Incorrect information in the HER (16%)
Electronic systems/technology failure (9%)	Hybrid health records/EHR conversion (15%)
Lack of EHR alert/alarm/decision support (7%)	Prepopulating/copy and paste (13%)
System failure—electronic data routing (6%)	EHR training/education (7%)
Insufficient scope/area for documentation (4%)	EHR user error (other than data entry) (7%)
Fragmented EHR (3%)	EHR alert issues/fatigue (3%)

Data compiled from Troxel, DB. Report: EHR-related malpractice suits have increased. https://www.thedoctors.com/search/?ssUserText=EHR-related+claims. Published October 10, 2017. Accessed October 18, 2017; and Cryts A. How to prevent malpractice lawsuits due to EHR errors. Medical Economics. http://medicaleconomics.modernmedicine.com/medical-economics/news/how-prevent-malpractice-lawsuits-due-ehr-errors?page=0,2. Published May 10, 2016. Accessed October 18, 2017.

basis. Formulate and record an updated Assessment and Plan each day based on current and relevant information. For more information, see Table 10-1.

IMPORTANT TIPS TO AVOID PROBLEMS

- Respect Health Insurance Portability and Accountability Act
- Be familiar with and follow compliance and ethics of your institution
- Avoid or disclose conflicts of interest
- Follow up orders, tests, and referrals: Close the loop
- Train staff to be helpful, not obstructive
- Report errors
- Obtain informed consent (procedures, transfusions, telemedicine, consultations, medications, everything) and document it
- Stay current—CME
- Check with your risk managers
- Standardized office/OR/rounding practices
- Team approach
- Bill appropriately

- Document, document, document
- Prepare, prepare, prepare
- Get good legal advice early and listen to it
- Be sure that your actions are well thought out and your defense reasoned
- Keep your cool and tell the truth
- Share only what you can remember or document
- You can never win at a deposition: but you can lose the case
- Be patient, be likeable
- Join a support group
- If your only concern is the welfare of your patients, it is unlikely you will be sued, and if you are sued, it is unlikely you will lose.

Figure 10-1 Actions practitioners may take if they are named in a lawsuit. From Peckham C. Medscape malpractice report 2015: why most doctors get sued. Medscape. http://www.medscape.com/features/slideshow/public/malpractice-report-2015#page=30. Published December 9, 2015. Accessed October 18, 2017.

CONCLUSION

The relationship between patient and provider is a sacred one built on trust, loyalty, and goodwill. Today's health care environment expects that we practitioners follow standards of best practice, use current resources, document carefully and honestly, and have near perfect outcomes. Sometimes, most practitioners will face a less-than-perfect outcome for his or her patient. These experiences are painful for both patient/family and practitioner. Being sued compounds the pain and may lead to self-doubt, humiliation, depression, fear of future patient encounters, defensive medicine tactics, and emotional/financial crisis.

This chapter presents some of the pitfalls that lead to medical malpractice lawsuits and suggestions on how to avoid them. If you are part of a medical malpractice suit, following here are some suggestions from a 2015 physician survey conducted by Medscape (Figure 10-1):

References

1. Jena AB, Seabury S, Lakdawalla D, Chandra A. Malpractice risk according to physician specialty. *N Engl J Med.* 2011;365(7):629-636.
2. Cornell Law School. Negligence. Legal Information Institute. https://www.law.cornell.edu/wex/negligence. Accessed October 18, 2017.
3. Rapp A. 10 simple tips to avoid malpractice claims. eMedCert. https://emedcert.com/blog/tips-to-avoid-malpractice-claims. October 6, 2014. Accessed June 10, 2018.
4. Bendix J. Your best malpractice defenses. *Medical Economics.* http://medicaleconomics.modernmedicine.com/medical-economics/news/your-best-malpractice-defenses?page=full. Published April 20, 2015. Accessed October 18, 2017.

Recommended Resources

Carrier ER, Reschovsky JD, Mello MM, Mayrell RC, Katz D. Physicians' fears of malpractice lawsuits are not assuaged by tort reforms. *Health Aff (Millwood)*. 2010;29(9):1585-1592.

Cornell Law School. Negligence. Legal Information Institute. https://www.law.cornell.edu/wex/negligence. Accessed October 18, 2017.

Cornell Law School. Tort. Legal Information Institute. https://www.law.cornell.edu/wex/tort. Accessed October 18, 2017.

Cryts A. How to prevent malpractice lawsuits due to EHR errors. *Medical Economics*. http://medicaleconomics.modernmedicine.com/medical-economics/news/how-prevent-malpractice-lawsuits-due-ehr-errors?page=0,2. Published May 10, 2016. Accessed October 18, 2017.

Diederich Healthcare. 2017 medical malpractice payout analysis. https://emedcert.com/blog/tips-to-avoid-malpractice-claims. Accessed October 18, 2017.

The Doctors Company. Interactive guide for electronic medical records. https://www.thedoctors.com/siteassets/pdfs/risk-management/interactive-guides/Interactive-Guide-to-Patient-Safety-for-Electronic-Medical-Records.pdf. Accessed October 18, 2017.

Gawande A. *The Checklist Manifesto: How to Get Things Right.* New York, NY: Metropolitan Books; 2009.

How to protect yourself from malpractice lawsuits. *Scrubs Magazine.* http://scrubsmag.com/how-to-protect-yourself-from-malpractice-lawsuits/. Updated January 13, 2017. Accessed October 18, 2017.

Murphy M. Steps providers can take to help avoid malpractice lawsuits. *Medical Scribe Journal.* http://scribeamerica.com/blog/steps-providers-can-take-help-avoid-malprac-tice-lawsuits/. Published October 7, 2014. Accessed October 19, 2017.

Peckham C. Medscape malpractice report 2015: why most doctors get sued. Medscape. http://www.medscape.com/features/slideshow/public/malpractice-report-2015#page=30. Published December 9, 2015. Accessed October 18, 2017.

11

Piles of Paperwork
Licensing, Certification, and Credentialing

Christopher A. Clyne, MD, MBA
Britton Jewell, DO, MHA

Becoming a licensed health care professional requires more than just completion of your training. Whether you wish to practice at a hospital or a clinic, you can count on a lot of additional paperwork to be required. Figure 11-1 summarizes the common components of maintaining licensure that are discussed in this chapter.

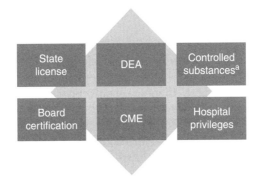

Figure 11-1 Common components of maintaining licensure. [a]See Appendix 2 for the list of states that require controlled substances registration. CME, continuing medical education; DEA, drug enforcement agency.

STATE LICENSE

You will need a separate state license for each state in which you wish to practice medicine. Each state has different requirements. For physicians, all states require completion of United States Medical Licensing Examination (USMLE) Step 3 or Comprehensive Osteopathic Medical Licensing Examination (COMLEX) Level 3. In some states, you can apply for licensure after completion of your internship year, whereas others require completion of the entire residency. Refer to Appendix 1 for the website information for each medical board, so you can contact them to determine the individual requirements.

DRUG ENFORCEMENT ADMINISTRATION REGISTRATION

The U.S. Department of Justice Drug Enforcement Administration (DEA) registration is required to prescribe controlled substances. You may apply for this online at www.deadiversion.usdoj.gov. If you practice at work sites (clinic, hospital, and office) in **different** states, you will need a DEA license for each state workplace address where you will be prescribing controlled substances.

CONTROLLED SUBSTANCES REGISTRATION

Refer to Appendix 2 for a list of states that require an additional controlled substances license in addition to the DEA registration. The address on the state-controlled substances license should match the address on the DEA registration.

BOARD CERTIFICATION

Many practice locations and employers will require you to be board certified or board eligible. Our recommendation is to take the board examination as soon as possible after the completion of your residency or fellowship because your knowledge base will be the highest. There are many opportunities for Board Review study guides, seminars, and review courses, both online and onsite. Refer to your organizational websites for scheduled courses/reviews and materials.

The American Board of Medical Specialties (www.abms.org) provides information on board certification for 24 different allopathic specialties. Osteopathic board certification information is provided at certification.osteopathic.org.

CONTINUING MEDICAL EDUCATION

In order to maintain your medical license and board certification, you will be required to complete continuing medical education (CME) activities. CME accreditation is adjudicated and implemented by the nongovernmental Accreditation

Council for CME. CME credits can also be required by hospitals to maintain credentialing and professional societies to maintain membership.

CME is important because it will help you stay up-to-date in your field and deliver the most effective care. There are thousands of CME activities held around the country each year. Requirements will vary by state and specialty board, but typically you will be required to complete around 50 CME credits annually to maintain privileges. Refer to Appendix 1 for the website information for each medical board so you can contact them to determine the individual requirements. Be sure to keep up-to-date on CME requirements and completion. Failure to complete these may jeopardize or delay the credentialing of privileges.

HOSPITAL PRIVILEGES

To admit and treat patients, you will need to apply for privileges at each hospital and recredential every 1 to 2 years. If you are self-employed, you will need to apply for them yourself. If you are employed, you will usually receive some assistance from a credentialing specialist and will have the appropriate paperwork sent to you. You may also apply for privileges for procedures you will perform in the hospital based on your specialty and expertise. Most hospitals and practices require documentation that you are adequately trained in the procedures for which you are asking to receive privileges. It is highly recommended that you keep a log of all procedures performed, especially for invasive techniques (eg, central line placement, lumbar punctures, catheterizations, sigmoidoscopies, bone marrow biopsies, intubations). Each completed procedure should be signed and dated by the preceptor for validation. It is also advisable to keep letters of recommendation on file so that they can be efficiently forwarded as needed to multiple sites.

INSURANCE APPLICATIONS

In order to bill insurance companies, including Medicare, Medicaid, and private insurance, you will need to fill out applications to be able to accept these insurances. If you are self-employed, you will need to apply for these yourself. If you are employed, you will receive assistance from a credentialing specialist. You may have already completed the appropriate paperwork when applying for hospital privileges.

OTHER CERTIFICATIONS

Many hospitals and other organizations may have additional requirements to maintain certifications such as Basic Life Support (BLS), Advanced Cardiac Life Support (ACLS), Advanced Trauma Life Support (ATLS), Pediatric Advanced Life Support (PALS), or National Institutes of Health (NIH) Stroke Scale. It is important to keep track of the expiration dates and renew them on time, especially if you are involved in running codes or responding to emergencies. Keep these certificates and dates for renewal in a file and calendar if possible.

Prescription Drug Monitoring Program

"Drug overdose deaths and opioid-involved deaths continue to increase in the United States. The majority of drug overdose deaths (more than 6 out of 10) involve an opioid. Since 1999, the number of overdose deaths involving opioids (including prescription opioids and heroin) quadrupled. From 2000 to 2015 more than half a million people died from drug overdoses. Ninety-one Americans die every day from an opioid overdose. We now know that overdoses from prescription opioids are a driving factor in the 15-year increase in opioid overdose deaths. Since 1999, the amount of prescription opioids sold in the United States nearly quadrupled, yet there has not been an overall change in the amount of pain that Americans report. Deaths from prescription opioids—drugs like oxycodone, hydrocodone, and methadone—have more than quadrupled since 1999."[1]

In an effort to prevent opioid overdose and abuse, clinicians are encouraged to follow practice guidelines for safe and effective treatment, such as those published by the Centers for Disease Control and Prevention (CDC). The CDC's guidelines for prescribing opiates for chronic pain can be found at https://www.cdc.gov/drugoverdose/prescribing/guideline.html.

To further reduce the opioid epidemic and related morbidity and mortality, every state except Missouri and the District of Columbia has a Prescription Drug Monitoring Program. You will need to contact the medical board of each state you are licensed in to be familiar with the rules and regulations requiring patient lookup when a controlled substances prescription is written. Refer to Appendix 1 for the website information for each medical board.

CERTIFICATION STORAGE AND SERVICES

It is highly recommended that a certification and credentialing file be created to store your letters, certificates, diplomas, awards, training, and licensure data for future reference because many states, institutions, hospitals, and practices will require individual application and credentialing.

In an effort to centralize the certification process, many states and organizations have adopted the Federation of State Medical Boards Federation Credentials Verification Service (FCVS) database/repository of medical education, postgraduate training, examination history, board action history, board certification, and identity. Physicians may use these stored data for medical licensure, hospital privileges, employment, or any number of legitimate agencies that accept FCVS as a valid primary source.

All states participate in the service. Some states require use of this service when applying for licensure; they are as follows:

- Kentucky
- Louisiana
- Maine—allopathic only
- Nevada—osteopathic only

- New Hampshire
- New York
- Ohio
- Rhode Island
- South Carolina
- Utah
- Wyoming

CONCLUSION

Owing to the large amount of applications, licensing, paperwork, verification, and references that are required to obtain privileges to practice in any state, it is our recommendation to allow at least 6 months for the entire process. Many hospitals and other practice locations will not even begin to process your application without a valid state license in hand first. You can easily add an additional 6 months to the process if you need to obtain a state license for the state in which you would like to practice first. Start the credentialing process as early as possible to avoid any gaps in your work history and potential loss of income.

Reference

1. Centers for Disease Control and Prevention. Understanding the epidemic. https://www.cdc.gov/drugoverdose/epidemic/index.html. Updated December 16, 2016. Accessed July 8, 2017.

Recommended Resources

Accreditation Council for Continuing Medical Education. For physicians and health care professionals. http://www.accme.org/physicians-and-health-care-professionals. Accessed July 8, 2017.

American Board of Internal Medicine. Procedural logbook. https://www.abim.org/~/media/ABIM%20Public/Files/pdf/publications/certification-guides/policies-and-procedures.pdf. Accessed July 8, 2017.

Federation of State Medical Boards. Federation Credentials Verification Service. https://www.fsmb.org/licensure/fcvs. Accessed July 8, 2017.

It Takes a Village
Social Work and the Community

Carla Martin, MD

INTRODUCTION

My career over two decades as a Meds/Peds physician has taken me to a variety of clinical settings, including community health centers, hospital wards, academic teaching clinics, urgent care centers, and private practice. A typical work day involves seeing 15 to 40 patients in the hospital or clinic: evaluating them, determining severity of illness, ordering diagnostic tests, and prescribing treatment plans.

As challenging as it is to care for such a large number of patients, my responsibilities as a physician used to be more well defined, and my training was more closely aligned with my practice. The practice of medicine has changed greatly over the past few years. Health care providers are now responsible for much more complicated care delivery.

An explosion of underinsured patients, drastically reduced funding to hospitals and practitioners, and a demand for improved quality of care and patient safety have taxed the clinical capabilities of practitioners who are also expected to be facile with many novel nonclinical responsibilities, such as electronic charting, insurance coverage nuances, and more complicated coding and billing practices.

Electronic health record (EHR) documentation, changing population demographics, and the Affordable Care Act's (ACA's) emphasis on providing health care in the communities and homes of patients rather than in institutions have all added to the complexity of successfully navigating the health care system for both patients and practitioners. One of my greatest challenges as a Med/Peds physician has been connecting patients of all ages and cultural and socioeconomic backgrounds to resources necessary for optimizing their health outside of the traditional medical structure (Figure 12-1).

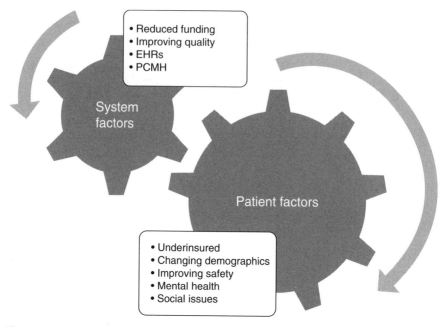

Figure 12-1 Challenges for the community medical practitioner. EHRs, electronic health records; PCMH, patient-centered medical home.

In view of the increasing complexity and demands of health care, and the interconnectivity made possible by an EHR, many delivery systems are moving to a team-based care model. Medical providers are trained to address patient's medical illnesses, but often not well trained to deal with psychosocial and mental health issues, including depression, anxiety, housing problems, addiction, food insecurity, abuse, and more. Many or all of these issues can be addressed by a nurse care manager, case worker, or social worker. You may be fortunate to work in a setting where you have access to a team of professionals to assist you in addressing these and other nonmedical issues that impact care, but if you do not, this chapter will help you prepare for some of these challenges.

THE "WHAT, WHO, AND HOW"

In order to provide the best care for our patients, practitioners must be familiar with the "What, Who, and How" of using community resources (Figure 12-2).

"What"—The Resources

The Patient-Centered Medical Home

The Patient-Centered Medical Home (PCMH) is a model for the provision of comprehensive and integrated care to patients of all ages. The goal is to establish

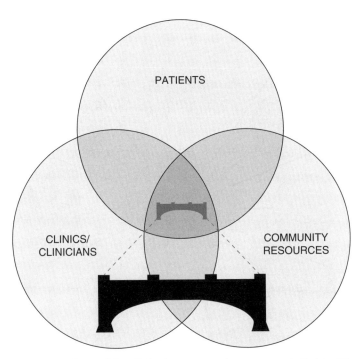

Figure 12-2 "What, Who, and How" of using community resources to "bridge" the gap between patients and providers. From the Agency for Healthcare Research and Quality Website. https://www.ahrq.gov/sites/default/files/wysiwyg/professionals/prevention-chronic-care/resources/clinical-community-relationships-eval-roadmap/evalfig.gif.

partnerships between the patients, the health care team, and sometimes the patient's family (especially pediatric patients). The practitioner provides continuous and comprehensive care to the patient together with a team that may include nurse care managers, nurses, medical assistants, pharmacists, social workers, behavioral health specialists, case managers, information technology experts, community health advocates, nutritionists, and more.

The patient is treated in the context of his or her economic and psychosocial situation, and it is the team's responsibility to connect the patient to other qualified professionals for acute, preventative, chronic, and end-of-life care as needed. Care is coordinated and integrated across the health care system that may link hospitals, specialty care, nursing homes, and community-based services. Enhanced access to high-quality, compassionate, and safe care is also part of the PCMH model. Ideally, there is shared decision making between the care team and the patient and patient's family.

This team model of care helps to alleviate some of the traditional tasks that providers had previously been doing (eg, medication reconciliation) and allows other team members to do screenings and enter data required for documentation into EHRs (eg, smoking status, diabetic foot exams, and drug and alcohol screenings).

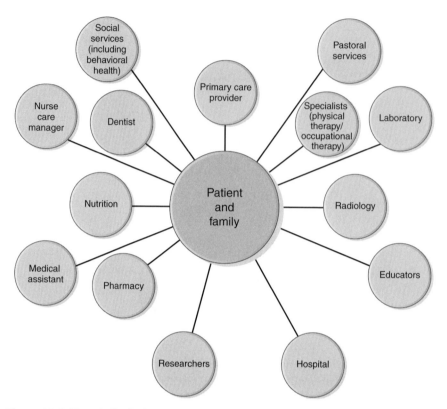

Figure 12-3 Many individuals/institutions involved in providing comprehensive patient care require a highly functioning, integrated approach to operate effectively.

The hope is that by having members of the health care team operate at the top of their respective licenses, clinicians can focus more on medical decision making, while limiting time spent on more tedious administrative tasks and allowing them to have a healthier work–life balance. The successful integration of a well-functioning team can improve job satisfaction, both for the clinician and other team members, while facilitating more comprehensive patient care (Figure 12-3).

Mental Health

Approximately one-quarter of American adults experience one or more mental health–related illnesses in their lifetimes. Many of these patients do not receive regular treatment in primary care practices, do not comply with treatment for their chronic medical conditions, and often end up in emergency rooms with higher acuity illnesses and higher cost of care.

One of the goals of the ACA was to provide better access to behavioral health services for patients in need. Medical providers often do not feel comfortable or adequately trained to provide mental health care. With a properly functioning team, the medical assistant can do a depression screening such as a Patient Health

Questionnaire-2 or anxiety screening such as a Generalized Anxiety Disorder-7. Positive screenings alert the clinician to further address the issue with the patient and appropriately treat and refer. The stress of chronic illness is itself a risk factor for mental health issues.

Most PCMHs have integrated behavioral health practitioners, such as a psychiatrist for medication management and/or a clinical social worker for psychotherapy. A licensed clinical social worker (LCSW) or a psychiatrist can often meet a depressed patient on the spot and help a medical practitioner assess whether a patient needs immediate hospitalization or can be managed as an outpatient with close follow-up. During a busy clinic day, one depressed patient who reports suicidal ideation can take a lot of time to properly triage.

Addiction

We have an opioid epidemic in the United States that will impact you in some way. Drug and alcohol use affects patient outcomes and has wide-ranging health and social consequences.

Medical conditions such as cardiovascular disease, stroke, cancer, HIV/AIDS, anxiety, depression, sleep problems, financial and legal difficulties, and work and family problems can all result from or be exacerbated by addiction.

In 2016, of the 8.9 million adults who have a substance abuse or mental health disorder, 37.6% did not receive any treatment (http://www.apa.org/helpcenter/data-behavioral-health.aspx).

Several screening tools are available to help assess who might benefit from treatment for drug or alcohol addiction. The Substance Abuse and Mental Health Services Administration and the Health Resources and Services Administration Center for Integrated Health Solutions promote integrated primary and behavioral health services. They provide training and assistance, and many screening tools are freely available on their website. The National Treatment Center Database allows one to search for addiction treatment centers by state.

Prescription Drug Monitoring Programs

A prescription drug monitoring program (PDMP) is an electronic database that tracks controlled substance prescriptions in a state. PDMPs can provide public health authorities with timely information about prescribing practices and patient behaviors that contribute to the epidemic. For practitioners, the databases help in assessing whether patients are compliant with their controlled medications and alert us to patients that may be diverting prescriptions.

This link can assist with finding a PDMP by state: https://www.cdc.gov/drugoverdose/pdmp/states.html.

Interpreter Services

Interpreter services are sometimes available through the patient's health insurance plan as well as through academic medical centers. The ACA has a requirement to provide interpreter services to patients of limited English proficiency.

Some practices have access to live interpreters or interpreter phone lines. Find out what interpreter service your site uses.

Arranging for an interpreter often requires advanced planning. In some states, for example, sign language interpreters have to be arranged at least 2 weeks ahead of time. If your practice does not have access to an interpreter service, you can search the National Board of Certification for Medical Interpreters at http://www.certifiedmedicalinterpreters.org/.

Some agencies can provide remote access to an interpreter through a phone line but may require a contract with your practice or health care organization before using their services. You may find some links through the International Medical Interpreters Association at http://imiaweb.org/.

Additionally, some medical schools offer basic medical language courses, which you will find helpful if you take care of a large population of foreign language–speaking patients.

Immigration

If you take care of immigrants and refugees, check with your city for social service agencies you can refer patients to. This immigrant services directory may be of some help: https://www.aclu.org/files/assets/ImServDir_20101229.pdf.

This is a listing with helpful links for immigrant families: https://www.childwelfare.gov/topics/systemwide/diverse-populations/immigration/helping-immigrant-families-overcome-challenges/.

The National Immigration Law Center can advise you about lawyers in your state certified to assist immigrants: https://www.nilc.org/.

Prescription Assistance

This organization has many useful links and information on their website for patients to assist with prescription medications, including a drug discount card for medications and medical supplies and links for participating $4 generic discount drug programs. It also has links where one can search by state for various programs, including low-cost clinics, dentists, transportation services, and government services: http://www.needymeds.org/.

Shelters

For links to shelters and transitional housing, visit at https://www.shelterlistings.org/.

Domestic Violence

The National Domestic Violence Hotline number to give to patients is 800-799-7233.

You can order cards to discreetly give to patients from many local domestic violence organizations. The website for the national hotline is http://www.thehotline.org/.

Reproductive Services

For women seeking reproductive services, Planned Parenthood is a resource: https://www.plannedparenthood.org/health-center.

Gun Violence

Gun violence has become a public health issue. Anticipatory guidance on gun safety to keep families safe is an integral part of a pediatrician's job. This pamphlet (from the Massachusetts Medical Society) is very useful in addressing this topic with your patients: http://www.massmed.org/uploadedFiles/massmedorg/Patient_Care/Health_Topics/Firearm%20Guidance%20for%20Providers%20final.pdf.

Public Health Departments and Medical Organizations

Familiarize yourself with your state's department of public health. It is likely you will interact with them for licensing, but they are also a resource for you. You may also contact your state's medical association, which often serves as an advocate for clinicians. Some states have a parent information network, which is especially helpful if you take care of families and children.

Table 12-1 lists other organizations that have chapters in many states:

This is a more extensive list of organizations providing health information: https://medlineplus.gov/organizations/all_organizations.html.

"Who"—The Professionals

Nurse Care Managers

Nurse care managers (NCMs) play an integral role in the PCMH. They focus on high-risk, complex, and resource-intensive patients within each office who are more at risk for emergency room visits and hospitalizations that drive up health care costs. They do much of the intensive care management of patients between visits with their providers. They maintain and adjust the patient care plan and engage patients with their care. They help evaluate their physical, mental, and psychosocial needs and serve as liaisons with other members of the care team and outside services, including visiting nurse association, wound care, and palliative/hospice services.

The NCMs ensure transitions of care such as rapid hospital follow-ups with reconciliation of medications and patient support. Their role is critical in caring for patients and helping to lower high-cost urgent and emergency care.

Social Workers

Social work is defined as "a community-based response to social need." Social workers help patients cope with the effects of social inequality such as poverty, illness, addiction, and domestic abuse. There are many things that affect a patient's

TABLE 12-1 Public Health Departments

The American Academy of Pediatrics
https://www.aap.org
345 Park Boulevard
Itasca, IL 60143
800-433-9016
The American College of Physicians
https://www.acponline.org
190 North Independence Mall West
Philadelphia, PA 19106-1572
215-351-2400
800-523-1546
The American Academy of Family Physicians
http://www.aafp.org/home.html
11400 Tomahawk Creek Parkway
Leawood, KS 66211-2680
800-274-2237
American Academy of Physician Assistants
https://www.aapa.org/about/
2318 Mill Rd., Street 1300
Alexandria, VA 22314
703-836-2272
American Association of Nurse Practitioners
https://www.aanp.org/
901 South MoPac Expressway
Building II, Suite 450
Austin, TX 78746

life and, ultimately, their health: income and poverty, cultural values, gun violence, and lack of adequate housing and food. Social workers can address these issues and try to assist patients in their own environment. They can provide case management (seeking and advocating for services for patients) and coordinate access to resources outside the provider's office.

Counseling and psychological interventions have also become part of the social worker's role. Social workers who earn degrees in clinical social work (LCSW), masters (MSW), or PhDs (DSW), often do individual psychotherapy, family, and group work in a variety of settings.

For help in finding a social worker in your community, you can contact the National Association of Social Workers. Their HelpStartsHere website offers a listing: http://www.helpstartshere.org/helpstartshere/?page_id=3677.

National Association of Social Workers
750 First Street, NE Washington, DC 20002
800-742-4089
https://www.socialworkers.org/

If you work in a practice without access to social workers, behavioral health, or nurse case managers, consider using a *toolkit* to determine and understand issues that might impact your patients' health, such as lack of adequate housing, food insecurity, and proper heating.

Health Leads has an excellent Social Needs Screening toolkit that can be downloaded from their website. It allows access to screening tools that are clinically validated. You can find the toolkit at https://healthleadsusa.org/tools-item/health-leads-screening-toolkit/.

Using a screening tool to address risk factors in patients who may be high utilizers can improve their health and also drive down overall health care costs by allowing you to appropriate resources to patients most likely to benefit from them.

Mental Health and Addiction Professionals and Resources

Some of the links discussed earlier will help you find resources in your community. Consider also searching for support groups, counselors, psychologists, and psychiatrists.

Your community's predominant health insurance companies may have a dedicated mental health customer service representative who can help patients find mental health providers who accept their insurance coverage.

The National Institute of Mental Health can provide some additional information: https://www.nimh.nih.gov/index.shtml.

This is the site for Alcoholics Anonymous to help you find a local chapter for your patients: http://www.aa.org/.

This is the site for Narcotics Anonymous: https://na.org/.

"How"—Accessing the Resources

Patient-Centered Hospital Transitional Care

Transitions of care, especially from hospital to outpatient, are vulnerable times for patients and are a risk for lapses in patient care, especially now that many primary care doctors no longer see patients in the hospital. It is important, if you are working in a hospital setting, to be aware of the discharge practices in your hospital both for better patient care and to avoid financial penalties from the Centers for Medicare and Medicaid Services imposed on hospitals for high readmission rates. Almost 20% of patients have an adverse event such as an infection, complications from procedures, and medication side effects within 30 days after discharge. These can be prevented with appropriate discharge planning. The transitional care from hospital to home or a facility such as rehabilitation or nursing home is the job of a team of providers that includes the bedside nurse, physicians or allied health professionals, discharge planner, and, sometimes, a patient advocate or social worker. The care planning team ensures that the patient and family are included in the discharge planning process. The patient and family should understand the diagnoses and treatment received in the hospital; and the discharge instructions, medications, and side effects should be reviewed; follow-up appointments made; and comprehensive discharge plans reviewed with patients and family members.

Patient Databases

Many states have databases that provide access to a patient's medications and medical problems from all sites as long as the patient is registered. These allow providers, for acute visits outside of the patient's medical home, to be able to obtain relevant information and connect with the primary provider. You can check with your local department of public health whether your state has this sort of program.

THE FUTURE

Medical teams will increasingly provide medical care for our population. It is necessary for health care practitioners to become familiar with each team member's role and background to optimize care of their patients. Ideally, medical and health profession students will be trained with more exposure to other disciplines and receive more education on team building. For example, at my local medical school, social workers help train medical students. This helps medical students early in their training become more aware of social needs and learn to work with allied health professionals.

As you strive to provide excellent care to your patients and connect them to resources, remember that sometimes what the patient needs the most is empathy. The video "Empathy: The Human Connection to Patient Care," produced by the Cleveland Clinic, is an excellent demonstration of this (https://www.youtube.com/watch?v=cDDWvj_q-o8).

Recommended Resources

Agency for Healthcare Research and Quality. IDEAL discharge planning overview, process, and checklist. https://www.ahrq.gov/sites/default/files/wysiwyg/professionals/systems/hospital/engagingfamilies/strategy4/Strat4_Tool_1_IDEAL_chklst_508.pdf. Published June 2013. Accessed November 29, 2017.

American Academy of Family Physicians. Joint principles of the patient-centered medical home. http://www.aafp.org/dam/AAFP/documents/practice_management/pcmh/initiatives/PCMHJoint.pdf. Published March 2007. Accessed November 21,2017.

American Psychological Association. Data on Behavioral Health in the United States. http://www.apa.org/helpcenter/data-behavioral-health.aspx. Accessed February 3, 2018.

Brearley J. *Counseling and Social Work*. Buckingham, UK: Open University Press; 1995.

Centers for Disease Control and Prevention. What States Need to Know about PMDPs. https://www.cdc.gov/drugoverdose/pdmp/states.html. Updated October 3, 2017. Accessed November 21, 2017.

Cochran J, Kenney CC. *The Doctor Crisis: How Physicians Can, and Must, Lead the Way to Better Healthcare*. New York, NY: PublicAffairs; 2014.

Emanuel E. *Reinventing American Healthcare: How the Affordable Care Act Will Improve our Terribly Complex, Blatantly Unjust, Outrageously Expensive, Grossly Inefficient, Error Prone System*. New York, NY: PublicAffairs; 2014.

Holland S, Scourfield J. *Social Work: A Very Short Introduction*. Oxford, UK: Oxford University Press; 2015.

Horwitz LI, Moriarty JP, Chen C, et al. Quality of discharge practices and patient understanding at an academic medical center. *JAMA Int Med*. 2013;173(18):1715-1722.

Johnson C, Houy M. Role of a nurse care manager in a patient-centered medical home: lessons learned from the Massachusetts patient-centered medical home initiative. *CMSA Today*. 2013;(2):8-11.

Jones A, Lemark CH, Lulias C, Burkard T, McDowell B, Severson K. Predictive value of screening for addressable social risk factors. *Journal of Community Medicine and Public Health Care*. 2017;4(2):030. http://www.heraldopenaccess.us/fulltext/Community-Medicine-&-Public-Health-Care/Predictive-Value-of-Screening-for-Addressable-Social-Risk-Factors.pdf. Accessed April 20, 2018.

Kern LM, Edwards A, Kaushal R. The patient-centered medical home and associations with health Care quality and utilization. *Ann Int Med*. 2016;164(6):395-405.

Kuzel AJ. Keys to high functioning office teams: trying to do it all yourself is not only unwise but increasingly impractical. *Fam Pract Manag*. 2011;18(3):15-18.

Merlino J. *Service Fanatics: How to Build Superior Patient Experience the Cleveland Clinic Way*. Philadelphia, PA: McGraw-Hill Education; 2015.

Sinsky CA, Willard-Grace R, Schutzbank AM, Sinsky TA, Margolius D, Bodenheimer T. In search of joy in practice: A report of 23 high-functioning primary care practices. *Ann Fam Med*. 2013;11(3):272-278.

Wachter R. *The Digital Doctor: Hope, Hype, and Harm at the Dawn of Medicine's Computer Age*. Philadelphia, PA: McGraw-Hill Education; 2015.

Carving Your Niche
Practice Paradigms

Christopher A. Clyne, MD, MBA
Britton Jewell, DO, MHA

Starting a new job is stressful. There are many things to consider and many changes, such as location, moving, housing, licensing and credentialing, and commuting. Perhaps the most important consideration for any health professional considering a new job is whether the position is a good fit. Are your skills and personality a match for the people and responsibilities of the new position? Will you be happy?

Being successful nowadays involves much more than just being a good doctor, practitioner, or administrator. In order to choose a job wisely and succeed, you must know the landscape (Figure 13-1):

- What kind of practice am I entering?
- Is the practice/company stable?
- What role will I play?
- How will I be compensated?

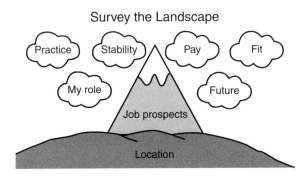

Figure 13-1 Many different factors to consider when looking for employment.

- Is this the right fit for me?
- What is my future here?

Health care has evolved over the past few decades from a majority independent/private practitioner fee-for-service model to one dominated by organizations and institutions. This metamorphosis is the result of the rapidly rising cost of health care with a focus on patient quality, safety, and efficiency.

Hospitals and health systems are shifting from a traditional volume-based to a value-based delivery system. Compensation is less based on volume. It is evolving toward a system that stresses quality, safety, and efficiency (lower cost). The Institute for Healthcare Improvement describes a "triple aim" design for improving and optimizing health care:

- Improving the patient experience of care (including quality and satisfaction)
- Improving the health of populations
- Reducing the per capita cost of health care

The result of this change has been a paradigm shift in the organization and practice of medicine.

The old model of one practitioner–one patient–one event is being replaced by a team approach to care for each patient longitudinally (lifetime) as part of a population. The patient/population will have access to a variety of services through the practice or institution. Reimbursement to the provider entity or entities from payers will be based on the outcomes of the individual and the population, such as expanded access, improved quality, and lower cost.

The success of provider systems (eg, hospitals, practices, health maintenance organizations [HMOs], individual practitioners) will also be linked to quality/safety, outcomes/access, and cost—the new triumvirate of health care.

There are few constants in this rapidly changing health care environment, but the practitioner driving clinical care is still the cornerstone of health care delivery. Success for the individual and the enterprise depends on a well-conceived and well-executed *alignment* of assets, goals, results, and incentives between practitioners and the practice/institution.

This chapter helps you to look beyond the compensation package alone and into the subtleties and nuances of what is involved in choosing the best practice paradigm for you.

We present and describe the many practice paradigm options and evolving landscape. It is important for practitioners, administrators, and consultants to be familiar with the forces of change because they will continue to color the practitioner's palate filled with the various complex practice paradigms (Figure 13-2).

REDUCE COST, IMPROVE EFFICIENCY

The cost of health care in the United States has been on a steady rise since the 1970s, currently consuming almost 18% of our gross national product. Small businesses that provide health insurance coverage for workers, and the individuals themselves, are seeing double-digit increases in premiums and rising deductibles.

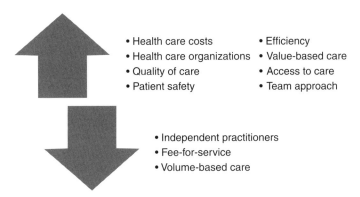

- Health care costs
- Health care organizations
- Quality of care
- Patient safety

- Efficiency
- Value-based care
- Access to care
- Team approach

- Independent practitioners
- Fee-for-service
- Volume-based care

Figure 13-2 Forces of change.

IMPROVE QUALITY, SAFETY, AND PATIENT SATISFACTION

This has always been a focus of health care, but became a priority and a target for measurement, improvement, and reimbursement after a 1999 report from the Institute of Medicine cited that there were between 44 000 and 98 000 annual deaths in the United States because of medical errors.[1]

The focus is no longer only on individual results, but on the overall outcomes of the entire population of patients in a practice.

WORK–LIFE BALANCE

Finding a position that makes room for one's priorities and interests outside of health care has become an important consideration for the new generation of practitioners and practices. Achieving balance enhances the satisfaction of the practitioner and the probability that the professional will be a long-term quality contributor to the practice and to their patients.

THE CASE FOR INTEGRATION/ALIGNMENT

These same forces have created a health care delivery system that is evidence based, data dependent, and compliance demanding. In order to provide quality care to large numbers of patients in a safe and efficient manner, practitioners and delivery entities (hospital and health care organizations) have found it advantageous to partner with each other. This has resulted in an *integration* and *alignment* of interests, skills, services, and resources that have completely changed the health care delivery paradigm.

GOALS OF ALIGNMENT

For Hospitals (Power in Numbers)

- Increase market share by aggregating practices and making alliances
- Manage cost through improved efficiencies and integration of services
- Improve quality and safety through standardization and sharing of resources
- Increase competitive advantage—for example, sharing of specialists among services
- Improve purchasing through group purchasing/bundling
- Enhance recruitment and contracting
- Enhance risk management/decrease medical malpractice insurance
- Unified strategic goals/planning
- Maximize revenue through pooled resources

For Practitioners (Safety in Numbers)

- Stabilize compensation in a decreasing market
- Decrease overhead and expenses (eg, labor, rent, and materials)
- Decrease administrative time/expense: billing, scheduling, credentialing, quality monitoring, and recruitment
- Reduce practice capital expenditures (eg, electronic health record [EHR])
- Ensure succession strategy: discourages "cash-out" option for senior members
- Increase technology and capital availability (eg, magnetic resonance imaging [MRI] and cath lab)
- Increase access to patients and new markets: promotion and marketing
- Maintain a role as a decision maker within the practice/institution
- Participate in new contract and compensation decisions, personnel decisions, governance, and acquisitions (eg, technology, buildings)
- Improve quality and efficiency through collaboration and integration
- Quality of life enhancement: work–life balance
- Maximize revenue through pooled resources

Figure 13-3 shows the benefits of alignment for the stakeholders involved.

PRACTICE MODELS

In essence, there are two major practice models: employed or independent (private). There are several varieties within each practice model. Becoming familiar with the models and their applications may help you to make the best decision when choosing a practice opportunity.

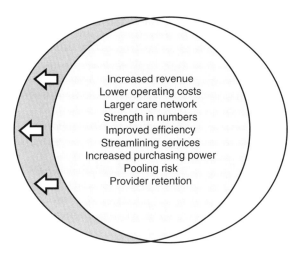

Increased revenue
Lower operating costs
Larger care network
Strength in numbers
Improved efficiency
Streamlining services
Increased purchasing power
Pooling risk
Provider retention

Figure 13-3 Alignment benefits.

Employed Practice Models

Fortunately, most practitioners are employed one way or another. The term "employed" here refers not to the arrangement that a practitioner has with the practice but to the autonomy of the practice.

An employed practitioner provides services exclusively for the organization and is bound by contractual provisions to the organization. The practitioner is usually compensated using a salary-based payment arrangement. Government health centers (eg, Veteran's Affairs, National Institutes of Health), HMOs, academic centers, hospitals, larger practices/clinics, and practice companies (eg, hospitalist companies, cancer centers) typically use this model.

The practice members understand that they are employees and not owners of the practice. Participation in policy, governance, and strategy decisions differs with each entity by contractual arrangement and may range from no influence to a rich collaboration.

Independent Practice Models

The alternative to working in an "employed" arrangement is to work for an "independent" or private practice. The success of any private or independent practice model in the modern era is successful integration of the practice with the hospital system or health care organization (eg, independent practice association, HMO, accountable care organization [ACO], and clinic).

Successful integration involves partnering with the organization's strategic goals, business practices, market opportunities, governance and administration, and overall culture. It is important for the private entity to be a "good fit" with the organization if a mutually beneficial relationship is to survive.

There are a number of independent practice models:

- Solo Practice: refers to one (or a few?) practitioner(s)
- Small Group General or Specialty Practice: for example, primary care physicians, cardiologists
- Large Group Single Specialty Practice: for example, large oncology or orthopedic surgery groups
- Multispecialty Practice: for example, cardiovascular group with noninvasive and invasive cardiologists, cardiovascular, and vascular surgeons

Figure 13-4 depicts these different types of practice models.

There are advantages and disadvantages of each type of practice model.

A SWOT (Strengths, Weaknesses, Opportunities, and Threats) analysis may be helpful to the practitioner in choosing whether to join an employed or independent/private group.

An example of a SWOT analysis for employment follows:

Strengths of Employment for the Practice/Practitioner:

- Income and benefits stability
- Decreased administrative duties
- Time management
- Advanced technology availability
- Access to larger markets
- Access to multiple specialties and resources

Weaknesses of Employment for the Practice/Practitioner:

- Limited autonomy in practice/business decisions
- Limited salary opportunity
- Limited involvement in governance and administration
- Productivity driven
- Large organizations often lack flexibility
- Impersonal/corporate culture

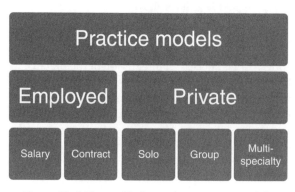

Figure 13-4 Types of independent practice models.

Opportunities for the Practice/Practitioner Through Employment:

- New market opportunities
- Access to new technologies
- Staff expansion
- Take advantage of competitor vulnerabilities
- Contract enhancements: directorships, bonuses, new products
- Service line development: shared resources
- Branding: as a member of a respected entity

Threats to the Practice/Practitioner Through Employment:

- Contract changes with insurer groups may limit access to some patients
- Competitor superiority may limit access to patients
- New administration may change partnering agreements, strategic goals, culture, and so on.
- Poor governance or management of the organization may impact practice's productivity and stability
- Straight salary/minimum: income guarantee or salary plus bonus/incentive (employed and private models)
- Equal shares: profits are shared equally (private model)
- Productivity based: as a function of how much you bring into the group or company (employed and private models)
- Capitated payment: a fixed fee is paid for each patient annually regardless of the amount or level of care received (employed and private models)

Figure 13-5 depicts this SWOT analysis for employment. There are several payment arrangements to fit the two models:

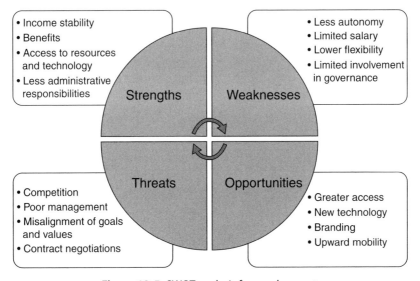

Figure 13-5 SWOT analysis for employment.

CURRENT AND FUTURE TRENDS IN MEDICAL PRACTICE

If there is a single term to describe the current trend in practice, it is alignment.

Internal forces for alignment include a shortage of physicians in many geographic areas; a shortage of specialists; a lack of interest in the administrative, regulatory, and financial burdens of running a practice by practitioners; reimbursement uncertainty by both parties; safer (improved?) earning potential for practitioners in a large organization; consolidation of resources increases efficiency (lowers cost); and demand for work–life balance.

External forces include competition from other entities for patients (market share) and talent (staff), loss of profitable revenue streams (eg, ambulatory centers, labs), increased governmental and nongovernmental (insurer) regulations requiring standardization (eg, EHR, best practices, quality reporting, "bundled" payments, and "shared" services), and increased capital expenditure requirements (eg, EHR, MRI scanner, compliance departments).

Figure 13-6 depicts these forces for alignment for stakeholders.

SPECTRUM OF ALIGNMENT RELATIONSHIPS: LOOSE–MODERATE–STRONG (EXAMPLES)

Loose alignment relationships include:

- Call coverage
- Medical directorships
- Managed care networks

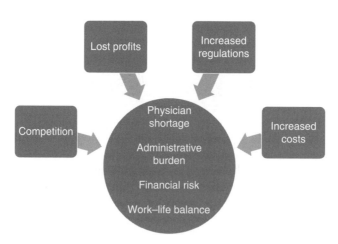

Figure 13-6 Forces for alignment.

TABLE 13-1   Practice Patterns From 2012 to 2016 Showing Movement Toward Employment Model

	2012	2014	2016
Practice owner	48.5%	34.6	32.7
Employed by hospital	43.7 (includes large group)	30.4	34.6
Employed by large group	No data	22.4	23.3
Other	7.8	12.5	9.4

Data From The Physicians Foundation. 2016 survey of America's physicians: practice patterns and perspectives. https://physiciansfoundation.org/research-insights/physician-survey. Published September 2016. Accessed January 3, 2018.

Moderate alignment relationships include:

- Service line management agreements: shared management of a service line (eg, cardiovascular service line)
- Comanagement arrangements: shared management
- Management service organization: hospital/organization manages parts of practice (eg, billing and collections, scheduling of patients and providers)

Strong alignment relationships include:

- Accountable Care Organization (ACO)/Clinically Integrated Network (CIN)[2]
- Professional service agreements: practitioner as an independent entity contracted to a hospital/organization
- Practice Management Agreements: hospital/organization manages entire practice
- Hospital or large group employment: the strongest relationship

The 2016 Physicians Foundation Survey published by Merritt Hawkins shows the state of alignment, with employment (vs private practice) leading the increasing trend since 2012 (Table 13-1).

CONCLUSION

External and internal challenges are forcing changes in how practitioners and administrators will participate in health care delivery in the United States. These forces are moving rapidly and are unpredictable in the current political and economic environment, making it difficult to know which practice model will be most advantageous and endurable.

Understanding the forces of change, the variety of practice models, and the benefits and risks of each model can help the practitioner and administrator to choose the practice that best fits their individual situation.

References

1. Institute of Medicine. *To Err Is Human: Building a Safer Health System.* Washington, DC: National Academies Press; 2000. Accessed January 3, 2018.
2. Tangible Solutions. CIN and ACO: What's the Difference? https://www.tangible.com/blog/value-based-care/cin-and-aco-whats-the-difference

Recommended Resources

The Physicians Foundation. 2016 survey of America's physicians: practice patterns and perspectives. https://physiciansfoundation.org/research-insights/physician-survey. Published September 2016. Accessed January 3, 2018.

From Bedside to Boardroom
The C-Suite

Christopher A. Clyne, MD, MBA
Britton Jewell, DO, MHA

We practitioners are more than just deliverers of health care. We are stewards of health care in the business of treating, maintaining, and preserving health for individuals and populations. The evolving priorities of American health care challenge us to become participants in the fiscal and operational aspects of health care. This chapter describes the opportunities, challenges, and attributes of the health care executive, how to become one, and what it means for the practitioner to be in health care administration.

The physician or practitioner usually makes the final decision about how care is delivered for the individual patient, but who makes the institutional decisions that will affect thousands of patients? Government, industry, academia, community, patients, businesses, and administrators are all stakeholders in American health care. This is a complex mix of often competing agendas and perspectives.

Over the past several decades, health care has become a huge industry, requiring those leaders of health care enterprises (eg, hospitals, health care organizations, and practices) to have an understanding of many things outside of medicine:

- Finance: Cash flow, profit and loss, balance sheets, income statements, payment reform, return on investment, investment (the long view)
- Ethics and Compliance: Culture
- Human Resources: Personnel
- Patient Satisfaction: Public relations (PR)
- Governance: Team
- Government Regulations and Policy: Regulations
- Social Media: Communication
- Technology: Data analytics

In our current system, administrators who may not have experience taking care of patients and may not have the full support of rank and file practitioners, often make these decisions. Physicians may have a better understanding of patient/population health care needs and have more support of practitioners "on the ground," but are not trained to run a business enterprise. Such endeavors are team dependent.

Administrators and boards of directors influence and create policy, implement procedures, and purchase technology and expertise (staff) that affect entire populations of patients. Physicians are trained to make individual patient care decisions based on data that are immediate and evidence based. Although consultation and collaboration among practitioners is frequent, the final decision is always an individual one between the patient and the provider. Physicians have not traditionally aspired to fill administrative/executive roles in administration or business that require a team approach with a "long-game" view of the vision and mission of the institution; but if we want to preserve our relevance and participation in making decisions about the Who, What, and How of health care delivery, we must become educated and engaged in the mechanics and administration of health care. There is no better place to do this than the "C-suite."

Health care dollars spent accounts for nearly 18% of America's gross national product. It is imperative that we learn to be lean and efficient to reduce cost if we are to provide first rate health care for our fellow citizens. This should not, however, be at the expense of quality, and no one understands what quality health care is better than those who deliver it on the ground every day. Government, hospitals, and patients are realizing that whatever business challenges exist for health care entities, an understanding of patient needs is paramount to running a successful health care organization. Physicians and nurses are also realizing that they can impact the care of entire communities by entering the "C-suite." Where there was little interest in hospital- and industry-related administration for practitioners, there is now an aligned interest in bringing the practitioner into the boardroom.

WHO IS IN THE C-SUITE?

- Chief Executive Officer (CEO):
  - Sets the vision ("who we are and what we want to achieve") and mission ("how we get there") of the enterprise (Figure 14-1).
  - Responsible for all aspects of the health care entity: financial/productivity, quality, personnel, PR, strategy and future planning (legacy), and operations.
  - Qualifications: MD/DO, Nursing, Attorney, and MBA/MHA.
  - Reports to board of directors.
- Chief Operations Officer:
  - Responsible for implementing all operations and strategic goals of the institution, including capital planning, staffing, mergers and acquisitions, facility planning, operational efficiencies (Six Sigma and Lean), and PR/community relations.
  - Qualifications: MBA/MHA.
  - Reports to CEO.

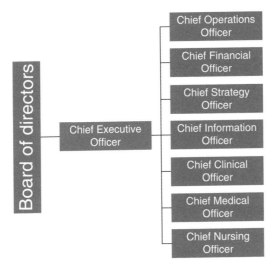

Figure 14-1 Structure of the C-suite.

- Chief Financial Officer:
  - Leads the institution in the effective deployment of capital toward improved financial performance.
  - Manages decisions about current and future revenue and debt and impact on the institution's financial health.
  - Responsible for all financial operations of the institution.
  - Qualifications: MBA.
  - Reports to CEO.
- Chief Strategy Officer:
  - Identifies opportunities for growth, partnership, and expansion of services by planning, guiding, executing, communicating, and sustaining the strategic goals of the institution.
  - Qualifications: MD/DO, Nursing, MBA/MHA.
  - Reports to CEO.
- Chief Information Officer:
  - Leads the institution in planning and acquisition of tools necessary for handling safe access to, and storage of, the massive amount of digital information available to practitioners, nurses, and other employees. Chief Medical Information Officer [CMIO]/ Chief Nursing Information Oﬁicer [CNIO].
  - Qualifications: BS, PhD, MD/DO, Nursing. MBA/MHA.
  - Reports to CEO.
- Chief Clinical Officer:
  - A member of the executive C-suite whose job is to drive physician alignment and the transformation of clinical care throughout the enterprise: strategy, communication, reimbursement experience, and leadership skills.
  - Roles may overlap with those of CMO.
  - Qualifications: MD/DO.
  - Reports to CEO.

- Chief Medical Officer/Chief Nursing Officer (CMO/CNO)
  - A hospital leader with both clinical and administrative/business credentials who acts as the hospital's representative to physicians/nurses.
  - Works closely together to ensure safety, quality, and productivity.
  - Responsible for influencing administration and medical/nursing staff to work together and find mutually beneficial alignments.
  - Qualifications: MD/DO, RN.
  - Reports to CEO.

ATTRIBUTES OF A HEALTH CARE EXECUTIVE

The health care executive must possess the attributes of any organizational leader (Figure 14-2):

- Independent thinker: Change leader
- Excellent listener: Collaborator/team player/empowers others
- Ability to influence, motivate, and inspire using knowledge and referent power and reputation
- Trustworthiness/transparency
- Organized planner who has a handle on all operations: Sets goals and measures results
- Excellent communication skills/tech savvy/PR
- Focuses on needs of staff, patients, and partners rather than on self

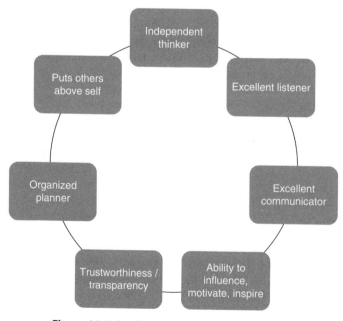

Figure 14-2 Attributes of a health care executive.

In addition to these leadership traits, the health care executive has a special calling to serve the ill and infirm, the community, and the public health at large. They must understand the stresses of being ill and the stresses of caring for the ill and dying. They must be a supporter of education and research because the quality of the health care product (personal and population health) is directly dependent on the advancement of research and dispersion of knowledge.

CHALLENGES FOR THE PHYSICIAN EXECUTIVE

"There is no 'I' in 'Team'. . . but there is 'm-e'"

Health care, like most large enterprises, moves slowly and takes time to adjust to new rules and change direction. Business leaders are trained to "see the big picture," to be patient, to ask, not tell. They rely on delegates and a team approach to accomplish the long-range goals of the institution. Theirs is a world of compromise and collaboration.

Physicians and other practitioners are not traditionally team players. We are trained to be autonomous and to micromanage. We are lone leaders trained to take control, analyze quickly, and make timely decisions based on readily available information: we select "right or wrong" diagnoses—black or white. There is little "gray" in medicine.

PRACTITIONERS LACK "ON-THE-JOB" BUSINESS TRAINING

Most doctors and other practitioners didn't choose medicine/health care so they could be leaders in administration. They prefer patient contact and dedicate massive amounts of time and energy to delivering care to individuals in need. There was little interest, and even less time, in training to be institutional leaders and businesspersons. Most practitioners lack the training in management and finance to be effective business leaders.

Leaders in the business setting are groomed for leadership through their work experiences over years with gradually increasing responsibilities and challenges, whereas practitioners have been shielded from the rigors and distractions of administration by focusing on the delivery of care. There has traditionally not been an effort to provide doctors and other practitioners with the necessary tools for leadership and the training to lead and provide long-term strategies for an organization. Leadership was opportunistic rather than planned for most physician leaders.

WHY PHYSICIANS AND PRACTITIONERS CAN BE GOOD LEADER-EXECUTIVES

Physicians and other practitioners are health care's "subject matter experts." As experts, they have the credibility and experience to set appropriate goals and create standards for care and mutually beneficial work environments. When these experts are put into the leadership roles of a health care entity, it sends the message to internal and external stakeholders that the institution's priority is the delivery of care. When a physician or practitioner is at the helm of a health care institution, it has been shown that there is more engagement of other practitioners. They relate to the leader as someone who has "walked the walk" and understands the stresses of the job.

Doctors and practitioners know what is needed to provide safe, quality care for their patients. What they often lack is knowledge and training in management, strategy planning, finance, and leadership. Many institutions are now working to provide leadership opportunities and training programs. There are currently two paradigms for transforming physician/practitioners into health care leaders (Figure 14-3).

Sharing Leadership: the Dyad System

The dyad system is a partnership between an administrative leader and a physician/practitioner leader who work closely together combining the skills and experience of each to forward the goals of the service line and institution. There is a true partnership in decision making: the administrator is an expert in management and finance, whereas the practitioner is an expert in patient care issues. By working together, they partner to create a service that can achieve the triple-crown goal of quality, safety, and reduced cost. In the process, each provides training and education for their counterpart.

The benefit of a dyad system is that it can provide the full range of expertise and services needed to run a successful health care enterprise. Additionally, it promotes (and indeed relies on) teamwork and trust between administration and practitioners.

This system has been successful for a number of hospitals, but like any system, there can be challenges, including power struggles, conflicting priorities, and personality differences. To be successful, the dyad structure requires clearly stated roles and goals and a willingness to share the leadership position—skills that are often lacking in physician leaders.

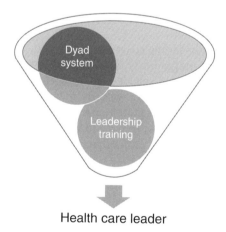

Health care leader

Figure 14-3 Practitioner/leadership paradigms.

Leadership Training

Tools Employed for Leadership Training

Most health care executive training programs recognize a sort of leadership ladder where an individual (future leader) learns more advanced leadership skills through a combination of coaching and graded responsibility—more complex leadership levels require different skills. Mastery of one level suggests the development of the necessary skills and understanding of the needs and goals of the organization, leading to higher levels of responsibility over time (Figure 14-4).

- Self-awareness/assessment tools (eg, 360°, Caliper)
- Consultants in long-range strategy formation, personnel, and financial management
- Executive coaching in communication and relationship building/collaboration
- Organizational leadership training programs for future physician/practitioner leaders (eg, Mayo Clinic, Cleveland Clinic, Kaiser Permanente)

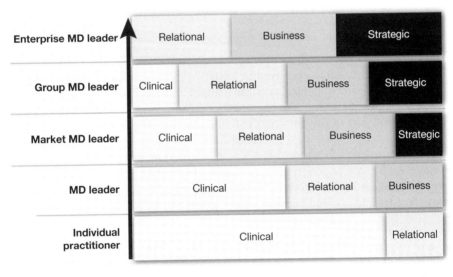

Figure 14-4 Physician leader skill requirements. Clinical: Delivery of patient care, including coordinating care and bedside manner/relational aspects of care delivery (vs business or operations management). Relational: Managing and developing others, including interpersonal skills, collaboration, and emotional intelligence/ behaviors. Business: Business management and administrative/operations (financial, operations, etc). Strategic: Setting goals, long-term direction, managing complexity. From Perry J, Mobley F, Brubaker M. Turning great doctors into great leaders: how healthcare organizations are boosting performance by building a pipeline of physician leaders. FMG Leading. https://static1.squarespace.com/static/5229fc34e4b0544e6521074b/t/59a5b3ad6f4ca3d5ae47c7cf/1504031678682/Turning+Great+Doctors+Into+Great+Leaders.pdf. Accessed March 16, 2018.

DO DOCTORS MAKE GOOD LEADERS?

Currently, only 5% of American hospitals are physician led, yet many believe that physicians have great potential for executive leadership because they are comfortable making important decisions, have "peer–peer credibility," and understand that patient needs come first and are the priority for an entity whose product is human health.

Domain experts—"expert leaders"—have been linked with better organizational performance in a variety of settings, including some of the nation's leading hospitals.

Physicians and practitioners are uniquely qualified to make patient-centered, value-based decisions for an institution. Studies support the role of the physician executive in leading hospitals to better organizational performance, higher employee satisfaction and engagement, and better safety and quality outcomes.

Organizations that have encouraged and empowered physician leaders have also shown healthier financial outcomes by making better value-based decisions and standardizing practices across service lines and practices.

SUMMARY

Health care is facing extreme challenges to expand access, improve patient quality and safety, and reduce cost. Finding leaders who can combine patient-centered clinical skills, business acumen, and leadership skills is necessary for the survival of a health care entity. There is an alignment of commitment to organizational leadership on the part of the physician/practitioners and recruitment on the part of the organizations. Health care enterprises recognize the need for physician/practitioner executive leaders and are providing executive training opportunities for physicians. An MBA is no longer a requirement to enter the C-suite. Recognizing and embracing these leadership opportunities is important to the success of the health care industry and can lead to a very fruitful career as a health care executive leader.

EDUCATIONAL RESOURCES FOR PHYSICIAN EXECUTIVES

If you want to build your executive skills, you can turn to a number of excellent sources of publications, seminars, and networking opportunities. Here are some of the best:

American Academy of Family Physicians

The American Academy of Family Physicians (AAFP) offers a Fundamentals of Management program. Over this year-long program, participants complete classroom work, an individual management project, and one-on-one consultation with an advisor. For more information, visit www.aafp.org/fom. The AAFP also hosts an Annual Leadership Forum in Kansas City, MO.

American Association for Physician Leadership

The American Association for Physician Leadership, formerly called the American College of Physician Executives, offers leadership and management courses designed for physicians. They offer the Certified Physician Executive designation for physician leaders who hold an advanced business degree and complete additional requirements. For more information, visit www.physicianleaders.org.

Medical Group Management Association

The Medical Group Management Association also offers conferences and seminars to physician and nonphysician managers. They offer several publications targeting medical group executives. For more information, visit www.mgma.com.

American College of Healthcare Executives

The American College of Healthcare Executives offers courses and many publications for health care executives. For more information, visit www.ache.org.

Society of Teachers of Family Medicine

The Society of Teachers of Family Medicine offers seminars and educational materials for family physician leaders in academic settings. For more information, visit www.stfm.org.

Recommended Resources

Angood P, Birk S. The value of physician leadership. *Physician Exec.* 2014;40(3):6-20.

Castellucci M. Teaching physicians how to lead. *Modern Healthcare.* http://www.modernhealthcare.com/article/20170325/MAGAZINE/303259983. Published March 25, 2017. Accessed March 16, 2018.

Mountford J, Webb C. When clinicians lead. *McKinsey Quarterly.* 2009. https://www.mckinsey.com/industries/healthcare-systems-and-services/our-insights/when-clinicians-lead. Accessed March 16, 2018.

Perry J, Mobley F, Brubaker M. Turning great doctors into great leaders: how healthcare organizations are boosting performance by building a pipeline of physician leaders. FMG Leading. http://www.fmgleading.com/blog/turning-great-doctors-into-great-leaders. Accessed March 16, 2018.

Stoller JK, Goodall A, Baker A. Why the best hospitals are managed by doctors. *Harvard Business Review.* 2016. https://hbr.org/2016/12/why-the-best-hospitals-are-managed-by-doctors. Accessed March 16, 2018.

Thomason S. Becoming a physician executive: Where to look before making the leap. *Fam Pract Manag.* 1999;6(7):37-40.

15

The Health Care Executive

Industry as a Career

Mark D. Carlson, MD

HISTORY OF PHYSICIANS IN INDUSTRY

Today, more physicians work in the medical device, medical technology, or pharmaceutical industry than ever before. Furthermore, physician career opportunities in these industries have never been more diverse. Established and start-up medical device, medical technology, and pharmaceutical companies seek and employ physicians in a variety of capacities and roles. As is the case with clinical practice, these roles provide numerous opportunities to improve patients' lives. In this chapter, we review some of the opportunities as well as the skills and characteristics that many companies seek in physician candidates for those positions (Figure 15-1).

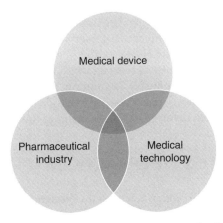

Figure 15-1 Career opportunities in areas of industry.

133

Today's biomedical technology companies employ physicians across a spectrum of functions, including medical affairs, clinical affairs (clinical study design and execution), regulatory affairs, research and development, safety (vigilance), education, business development (licensing, mergers, and acquisitions), and legal affairs. Physicians may begin their careers with these companies directly after graduating from medical school, after completing postgraduate education (residencies or fellowships), or later after having practiced medicine for many years. Not surprisingly, the positions available and the career paths that follow vary, depending on when one joins industry and the type of company (start-up vs established, pharmaceutical vs medical device) one joins.

EARLY CAREER OPPORTUNITIES

I am, with increasing frequency, engaged by physicians who ask about joining industry, sometimes very early in their careers or even immediately following completion of postgraduate training. As a general rule, the value of a physician to a company is commensurate with that individual's subject matter knowledge and experience practicing medicine. Whereas the MD degree provides a perspective that adds value, it alone does not differentiate the physician to the extent that years of clinical practice and clinical research experience do. However, there are entry-level and sometimes middle management positions for which physicians who have not practiced medicine may qualify. Early career physicians are sometimes employed in clinical affairs to design or manage studies; regulatory affairs to assist in gaining product approval; or postmarket surveillance, research and development, or safety. Physicians applying for these positions are often competing against individuals from adjacent fields who are more commonly employed in these positions (eg, nurses, biomedical engineers, statisticians). Whereas the medical degree confers certain advantages with regard to knowledge of diseases, diagnostics, and therapies, nonmedical candidates may have specific training and experience that is valued as well (eg, statistics, clinical study design, regulatory experience). Furthermore, a physician beginning a career in these disciplines can expect to follow a career path similar to a person without a medical degree or particular subject matter expertise. However, the pharmaceutical industry tends to employ physicians earlier in their careers and with less medical specialty training than does the medical device industry. In addition, start-up companies sometimes employ early career physicians, particularly if that individual has a strong research background and has been involved in development of the company's product.

OPPORTUNITIES FOR PRACTICING PHYSICIANS

Companies derive value in many ways from experienced practicing physicians. These individuals can provide insights into the unmet needs in a particular therapeutic area, identifying the needs of patients and physicians (problems worth solving) that may inform innovation and product development. They may assist in research and clinical study strategy, design, and execution. Practicing physicians may assist in product development in preclinical laboratory testing and may help guide development of innovative technologies being prototyped. They may advise on product performance and safety as well as identify ways to communicate such information to physicians, regulatory agencies, and the public. Companies often engage experienced practicing physicians as consultants (individually or in boards or committees) to gain their input. However, because the need for ongoing consistent clinical input has increased, companies have recognized the need for dedicated and readily available medical advice and leadership. Increasingly, companies have established medical affairs organizations populated by physician medical directors, nurses, and scientists, and led by chief medical officers or sometimes by nonphysician scientists.

Medical affairs organizations are most often led by a physician (chief medical officer) and, in larger companies, usually include additional geographically based and/or functionally oriented physicians (medical directors). Medical directors often work with others (eg, scientists, nurses, engineers) who extend the reach of the medical director and the organization by working closely under the direction of the medical director with key physician customers and investigators. The medical affairs organization typically adds value, in part, by providing a clinical and medical perspective that influences company decision making, among the functions noted earlier. In addition, medical affairs physicians and personnel interact with physician key opinion leaders, study investigators, and customers across a number of topics, including product performance, study design and execution, presentations and publications, and education and training. Medical affairs is generally independent of marketing and the commercial (sales) organization, which enables its personnel to provide information that focuses on science, is supported by the medical literature, or is based on clinical experience. Medical affairs physicians generally have credibility with their peers and colleagues because of their clinical experience and because they are known to and respected by their practicing physician colleagues.

The value of a chief medical officer or medical director to a company is derived largely from one's experience, relationships, and, as a result, ability to influence others and impact the medical community that is directly involved with products or technologies manufactured by the company. These characteristics are chiefly developed not only during medical training but also as the result of the experiences derived over a career in medical practice. Whereas medical training and clinical experience are a prerequisite, other skills, particularly communication and presentation skills, are required to excel as a medical director or chief medical officer.

A medical director typically has practiced her or his specialty for several years, is internationally known and respected, and has excellent listening and communication skills. Whereas the medical director is typically an expert in a particular field, he or she must set ego aside and listen to physician colleagues and other caregivers to understand their issues and point of view and to effectively influence clinical practice. The words of television talk show host Larry King apply: "I never learned anything when I was talking."

An effective medical director works collaboratively and collegially with company personnel across functions and at all levels. The ability to work in a team is critical to success; the medical director must understand that his or her opinion and perspective, although very important, is one of many that influence company decisions. An effective medical director knows what he or she knows and, more importantly, knows what he or she does not know.

CHALLENGES

Physicians (myself included) contemplating industry careers often express uncertainty regarding two questions: (1) How will I be compensated? and (2) What happens if it doesn't work out; will I be able to return to practice? These concerns tend to be greater among midcareer physicians than among those who contemplate working in industry either early or late in their career.

Financial compensation in industry is sometimes very different than in practice, particularly if the physician were in a practice in which there is no component of salary at risk or related to performance-based incentives. Typically, industry compensation includes a fixed base salary and several other components that vary based on both company and individual performance, including a bonus, equity, profit sharing, and sometimes a pension. The latter two are less common today than in the past. Typically, the base salary in industry is not commensurate with that of a practicing physician. It is the upside potential of the variable components that adds value and is sometimes the most difficult for physicians to grasp.

Physicians being considered for medical director/chief medical officer positions are usually at the peak of their practicing careers. Many are not looking for a career change; they enjoy what they are doing. It is no surprise that these physicians may be anxious to stop practicing medicine "cold turkey." In addition, they may have doubts about whether they will enjoy working in the company or whether they will succeed, because the roles and responsibilities of a chief medical officer are often very different from that of a practicing clinician. Finally, physicians recruited to medical affairs positions may be concerned about remaining clinically relevant, maintaining expertise and peer recognition that enable them to continue to be effective in their company role or return to practice. Hence, physicians considering these roles often voice interest in continuing to practice part time or episodically. Such arrangements vary in their logistics, complexity, and value to both the company and the physician employee and are often the function of the particular field of medicine and therapy area/product line in industry. Some physician specialties lend themselves to part-time clinical work; others do not. Some company positions allow time and derive value from the physician employee performing part-time clinical work; others do not. When I joined St Jude Medical in 2006, I had questions and concerns about stepping away from the practice of medicine. The chief executive officer (CEO) told me, "Your desk will be full on day one; you won't be bored." He was correct. Although I was allowed to continue to practice part time, I never did so. I have found, both for myself and for my physician colleagues, that concerns about stopping practice dissipate quickly after we engage our new industry position. There is too much to learn and there are too many interesting things to do, to dwell on it.

CAREER PATH

Some companies derive value from providing physician employees with opportunities in other disciplines during their career. For instance, a physician, initially hired as a medical director, might be asked to participate in, or even to lead, education and training or safety. Such experiences provide the physician with a broader perspective as well as business and management experience that can prepare them for future leadership opportunities. Such roles and opportunities often give the physician unique opportunities to engage with products, technologies, and fields of medicine outside of their area of "expertise" and offer the individual challenges that are valuable for individual growth.

Business development (eg, licensing, mergers and acquisitions) is a discipline that can benefit significantly from medical input because physicians often have unique insights regarding the potential benefits or limitations of a particular product or service. These insights are an important input, along with others (eg, intellectual property strength, manufacturing costs, competitive environment), that influence a company's business development decisions. Companies often gain these insights from physicians in the medical affairs organization and sometimes from physician consultants. Occasionally, physicians with strong medical and business skills may join or even lead a business development organization.

Physicians are increasingly included in the C-suite, either as a corporate chief medical officer or, sometimes, as the company leader. These leaders have often undergone formal business training and have experience managing a profit and loss sheet. It is not unusual for the physician founder of a start-up company to ultimately continue as the company's CEO. Physician CEOs of established companies tend to have significant industry experience and proven leadership skills.

How does a physician become a company leader? The answer begins with an understanding of what the company seeks (Figure 15-2). This may include any of the following:

- Relationships, recognition, and respect
- Medical expertise
- Research expertise
- Innovation expertise
- Product development expertise
- Listening skills
- Collaborative skills
- Business knowledge and experience

The first three (relationships, recognition, and respect; medical expertise; and research expertise) are interrelated and require career experience and demonstrated excellence following medical training. Proof points for these include participation and

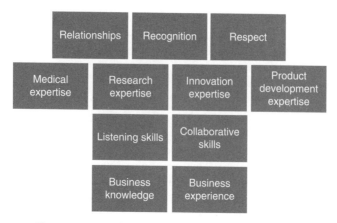

Figure 15-2 Attributes of a physician leader in industry.

leadership in clinical trials, publication and podium presence, medical society leadership experience, and public policy experience. Innovation and product development expertise may be exhibited through intellectual property development (patents) and/or previous work in or with other start-up companies. Communication and collaborative skills are less easily documented but are equally, if not more important, than many of the other qualifications. Companies pay great attention to these qualities when considering candidates. Hiring an experienced physician is a considerable investment for a company and is associated with significant risk because the implications of a failed physician hire go far beyond the lack of return on the investment.

There are two main professional societies for physician and other health care executives, namely, the American College of Healthcare Executives (ACHE; www.ache.org) and the American Association for Physician Leadership (AAPL; www.physicianleaders.org). The ACHE is open to all health care leaders and executives, regardless of their clinical backgrounds (or lack thereof). The organization offers a fellowship, Fellow of the American College of Healthcare Executives (FACHE), for board certification in health care management. The AAPL is open to physician leaders and executives and offers the certified physician executive designation awarded by the Certifying Commission in Medical Management. For more information on either organization, please see their respective websites.

CONCLUSIONS

Physician career opportunities in the biomedical technology industry are more prevalent and diverse than ever before. Meaningful opportunities exist for early, mid-, and late career physicians to impact companies and the physicians as well as patients they serve. A key to securing a position and to one's success thereafter is to understand clearly what the company seeks and to ensure that one's goals are aligned with those of the company. An industry career can be very rewarding in that it can enable a physician to impact the practice of medicine and the lives of multitudes of patients worldwide.

16

The Game Changer
The Affordable Care Act and Its Future

Christopher A. Clyne, MD, MBA
Britton Jewell, DO, MHA

The Patient Protection and Affordable Care Act (also known as the Affordable Care Act [ACA] or Obamacare) was signed into law on March 23, 2010, by President Barack Obama. This was a groundbreaking piece of legislation that fundamentally changed the US health care system. Despite numerous challenges by the states, Supreme Court cases, and opposition by Republican members of Congress and President Donald Trump, the ACA has not been completely repealed or replaced. Large volumes could be written about the ACA; however, this chapter focuses on the law's major provisions and the effects that it has had on the business of medicine.

MAJOR PROVISIONS OF THE AFFORDABLE CARE ACT

The ACA could be summed up as follows: The ACA sought to provide affordable health insurance coverage to all Americans, regardless of their ability to pay (Figure 16-1). Whether the law was successful in doing so has been the subject of constant debate. As of early 2016, the ACA has been successful in providing health insurance coverage for 20 million Americans. There are many ways in which the law sets out to accomplish this:

- Individual mandate
- Employer mandate
- Medicaid expansion
- Medicare improvements
- Premium subsidies

139

- Tax changes
- Health insurance exchanges
- Benefits package requirements
- Cost-savings measures
- Quality incentives
- Preventive services
- Long-term care programs

Individual Mandate

The ACA requires all individual citizens and legal residents to obtain qualifying health insurance coverage. If they do not, they are subject to paying a penalty tax. For 2016 and beyond, the tax penalty is $695 or 2.5% of income, whichever is greater. After 2016, the penalty was to be adjusted annually based on the cost of living. On December 22, 2017, the Tax Cuts and Jobs Act was passed, which repealed the individual mandate. This will not go into effect until 2019. It is unclear how this repeal will ultimately affect premiums, deductibles, subsidies, and coverage.

Employer Mandate

Employers that have 50 or more full-time employees and have at least one employee who receives a premium tax credit must offer health insurance coverage. If employers have more than 200 employees, they must automatically enroll them into a health insurance plan with the option for the employee to opt out.

Medicaid Expansion

The ACA expands Medicaid coverage greatly, making non–Medicare-eligible individuals younger than 65 years eligible for Medicaid if their adjusted gross income is up to 133% of the federal poverty level. Each state had the option of

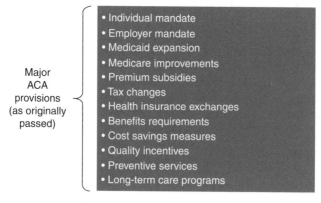

Figure 16-1 Major Affordable Care Act (ACA) provisions, as originally passed.

expanding its Medicaid coverage. As of January 1, 2017, 19 states have opted not to expand their coverage. Figure 16-2 shows which states have adopted, or not adopted, the Medicaid expansion.

States that chose to expand Medicaid received 100% federal funding to finance the cost from 2014 to 2016. For 2017, they received 95% federal funding. For 2018, they will receive 94% federal funding; for 2019, 93%; and for 2020 and beyond, 90%. Also, Medicaid rates for primary care physicians were increased to 100% of the Medicare rates for 2013 to 2014 with 100% federal funding. This made accepting ACA/Medicaid patients more reasonable for primary care physicians, who were often unable or unwilling to accept Medicaid patients because of the net financial loss the practice often had to absorb.

Medicare Improvements

The coinsurance rate for the Medicare Part D coverage gap (the donut hole) will be decreased from 100% to 25% by 2020. While in the coverage gap, generic drugs will be subsidized up to 75%, and brand name drugs will be subsidized

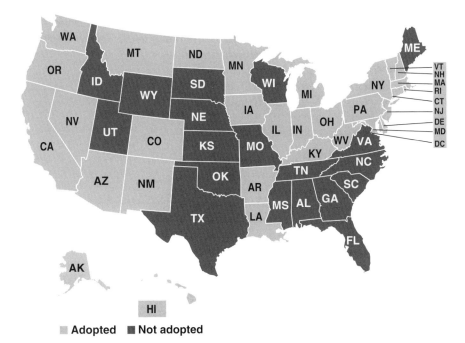

■ **Adopted**   ■ **Not adopted**

Figure 16-2 States that have adopted the Affordable Care Act Medicaid expansion. From Kaiser Family Foundation. Status of state action on the Medicaid expansion decision. The dark states are the ones that did not expand Medicaid. https://www.kff.org/health-reform/state-indicator/state-activity-around-expanding-medicaid-under-the-affordable-care-act/?activeTab=map&currentTimeframe=0&selectedDistributions=current-status-of-medicaid-expansion-decision&sortModel=%7B%22colId%22:%22Location%22,%22sort%22:%22asc%22%7D. Accessed April 20, 2018.

up to 25% by 2020. Brand name drugs are discounted by 50% starting in 2011. (For an explanation of the "donut hole," or coverage gap in Medicare Part D before and after the ACA, please visit https://blog.medicare.gov/2010/08/09/what-is-the-donut%C2%A0hole/.)

The amount of Graduate Medical Education slots (residency positions) was increased, prioritizing primary care and general surgery, and underserved and rural areas in an attempt to expand access.

SUBSIDIES

Individual and Family Subsidies

The ACA provides premium credits to individuals and families with incomes from 100% to 400% of the federal poverty level to help cover the cost of health insurance plans purchased through the health insurance exchanges. There are four types of metal plans determined by the relative premium amount the individual (low to high) or insurance company (high to low) pays: bronze, silver, gold, and platinum. The premium credit amounts are based on the cost of the second lowest silver plan offered in the area. The amount of premium credits received will vary based on income and decreases as income increases.

The ACA also provides cost-sharing subsidies to individuals and families with incomes from 100% to 400% of the federal poverty level to help cover out-of-pocket costs, such as deductibles and copayments, and lower the out-of-pocket maximum.

Employer Subsidies

Small employers with less than 25 employees and average annual wages of less than $50 000 are provided with a tax credit. Starting in 2014, if coverage was purchased though the health insurance exchange, the employer was provided with a tax credit of up to 50% of their contribution toward their employee's premium if they covered at least 50% of the total cost. This credit can be claimed for two consecutive tax years.

Tax Changes

The individual mandate (which was repealed as a part of the December 2017 Trump Tax overhaul) imposed a tax penalty of $695 or 2.5% of income, whichever was greater, for individuals without qualifying health insurance coverage. Over-the-counter drugs, not prescribed by a provider, were not to be reimbursed from a health flexible spending account (FSA) or a health reimbursement arrangement, or be reimbursed tax free from a health savings account (HSA). The distribution tax from an HSA for funds not used for qualified medical expenses was raised to 20%. FSA contributions were limited to $2500 per year starting in 2013, and were to be increased yearly by the cost of living. The limit for unreimbursed medical expenses included on income tax itemized deductions was increased to 10% of adjusted gross income. The Medicare Part A tax on wages was increased from 1.45% to 2.35% in 2013, for individuals making more than $200 000 annually and $250 000 for joint filers. In addition, a 3.8% tax was to be applied to unearned income for filers above these thresholds. In 2020, an excise tax, also known as a Cadillac tax, of 40% was to be imposed on insurers for plans with premium costs greater than $10 800 for individual and $29 100 for family plans. Pharmaceutical manufacturers were subject to annual fees of $4.0 billion in 2017, $4.1 billion in 2018, and $2.8 billion in 2019 and beyond. Health insurers were subject to annual fees of $13.9 billion in 2017 and $14.3 billion in 2018. For 2019 and beyond, the fee would be increased from the previous year's by the rate of increases in premiums. Medical device sales were subject to a 2.3% excise tax. Indoor tanning services were subject to a tax of 10%.

Health Insurance Exchanges

The ACA created individual and small business health insurance exchanges to allow individuals and small businesses to purchase qualified health insurance coverage. An exchange dedicated to enrolling small businesses is called a Small Business Health Options Program Exchange. In each exchange, at least two multistate plans must be offered, at least one plan must not cover abortions (except those permitted by federal law), and at least one plan must be offered by a nonprofit organization. The Consumer Operated and Oriented Plan program was created to encourage nonprofit, member-run health insurance companies to offer qualified plans on the exchanges and was funded with $4.8 billion.

The exchanges must provide five different types of plans: bronze, silver, gold, platinum, and a catastrophic plan. The "metal" plans provide essential health benefits and cover a portion of the benefit costs (bronze—60%, silver—70%, gold—80%, platinum—90%). Catastrophic plans are an option for individuals up to age 30 or for those who are exempt from the individual mandate, and only provide catastrophic coverage. All of these plans are subject to an out-of-pocket maximum that equals the HSA limit, which was $5950 for individuals and $11 900 for families in 2010. The out-of-pocket maximum is limited for individuals/families with incomes from 100% to 400% of the federal poverty level (one-third of the HSA limit for 100%-200%, one-half of the HSA limit for 200%-300%, and two-thirds of the HSA limit for 300%-400%).

The plans offered on the exchanges must only change their premiums based on age, family composition, premium rating area, and tobacco usage. A permanent risk adjustment program was created, which provides payments to insurers based on the "risk" of their members and on their demographic information and health status. Lower risk plans must provide payments to higher risk plans in order to "equalize" the risk-benefit for the insurer.

BENEFITS PACKAGE REQUIREMENTS

The ACA requires all individual and small group plans to offer an essential health benefits package, whether offered through the exchanges or not. This package includes 10 different categories:

- Ambulatory patient services
- Emergency services
- Hospitalizations
- Newborn and maternity services
- Behavioral health, mental health, and substance abuse treatment
- Prescription drugs
- Rehabilitative and habilitative devices and services
- Laboratory services
- Chronic disease management, preventive and wellness services
- Pediatric services to include vision and dental care

The exact essential health benefits package varies from state to state and from year to year. The plans may differ in coverage of certain benefits, coverage limits, and prescription drugs. The ACA prohibits abortions from being a required part of the essential health benefits package.

PRIVATE INSURANCE CHANGES

- The ACA provides standards to lower administrative costs: The ACA requires health insurers to maintain a medical loss ratio of 85% for large group market plans and 80% for individual and small group market plans. The medical loss ratio is the proportion of premium revenue spent on providing care and quality improvement relative to administrative costs. If administrative costs are above this threshold, the insurer must provide a rebate to its members.
- Increases in plan premiums must be reviewed and must be justified by the insurer. The states must track increases in premiums and may recommend that certain plans be barred from the exchanges because of rate increases.
- All individual and group plans must continue dependent coverage up to age 26. Additionally, these plans cannot place lifetime limits or annual limits on the amount of coverage. Coverage cannot be taken away except for fraud.
- Preexisting condition exclusions are eliminated. All new plans must be in line with one of the four "metal" plan categories. Small group market plan deductibles must be limited to $2000 for individuals and $4000 for families. Waiting periods before coverage begins is limited to 90 days.
- A temporary reinsurance program was created to provide funding to insurers that enrolled high-risk (and high-cost) individuals. This program was active from 2014 to 2016 and was funded from all health insurers at a total cost of $25 billion.

- The ACA created standards for how plan information is to be given to individuals and provided for the creation of a website to determine coverage options.
- The Health Insurance Reform Implementation Fund was created to distribute $1 billion to carry out health reform policies.

COST-SAVINGS MEASURES

Health insurers must utilize administrative simplification requirements to control costs, such as applying a single method to determine eligibility, claims status, payments, enrollment and disenrollment, electronic funds transfers, and referrals, or be penalized no more than $1 per member.

Medicare Advantage (MA) plans are required to maintain a medical loss ratio of 85%. MA payments were redistributed to lower costs, based on the Medicare fee-for-service rates. Payments were increased in areas with low fee-for-service rates and decreased in areas with higher fee-for-service rates. Plans with four or more stars (out of five) were given bonuses, starting in 2012. Rebates were also adjusted based on this quality score.

The Medicare annual market basket update (https://www.cms.gov/Research-Statistics-Data-and-Systems/Statistics-Trends-and-Reports/MedicareProgram-RatesStats/downloads/info.pdf), an adjustment to reimbursement based on the increase in costs of goods and services, was reduced and adjusted based on productivity for inpatient hospital, skilled nursing facility, home health, hospice, and other Medicare providers. The ACA created a productivity adjustment factor that decreases the market basket update based on a presumed increase in efficiency of health care workers, which should increase productivity. This productivity adjustment has been estimated to decrease the market basket update by 1.1%, on average. This adjustment serves as a mandate for increased efficiency.

The Medicare Part B income-related premium thresholds are frozen until 2019 and will not rise with inflation. The Medicare Part D premium subsidy is reduced for incomes greater than $85 000 for individual and $170 000 for joint filers.

An Independent Payment Advisory Board (IPAB) was created to make recommendations to reduce Medicare spending if it exceeds certain thresholds. Starting in 2015, this Board must make recommendations every other year to decrease the health care costs. Starting in January 2018, the threshold is reached if Medicare spending is greater than gross domestic product plus 1%. The IPAB consists of members of industry, government, business, economics, academia, and health care for 5-year appointments by the Executive branch. It does not permit any practicing physician to be on the Board.

An Innovation Center was created to assess new payment models to lower costs and improve quality for Medicaid, Medicare, and the Children's Health Insurance Program.

The Medicare Disproportionate Share Hospital (DSH) payments are first decreased by 75%, and then increased by the number of uninsured patients and free care given. DSHs are those that have a large number of uninsured, low-income, and Medicaid patients. Medicaid DSH payments are reduced by $1.8 billion in 2017, $5 billion in 2018, $5.6 billion in 2019, and $4 billion in 2020. The deficit in DSH payment for uninsured was to be offset by the increased numbers of ACA insured Americans.

Accountable care organizations (ACOs) can receive some cost sharing that they realize in providing care for their Medicare patient population. ACOs are so named because they are "accountable" for the care they provide. They must have measures in place to report on their costs, quality, and coordinate care, and have suitable primary care provider involvement.

Medicare payments are reduced to hospitals for hospital-acquired conditions by 1% and are also reduced for preventable readmissions. Federal Medicaid payments to the states are reduced for health care–acquired conditions such as catheter or surgical infections.

Every 3 years, nonprofit hospitals must perform a community needs assessment. This includes an execution strategy tailored to the community's needs and a financial assistance policy.

There are many different initiatives to decrease waste, fraud, and abuse, such as creation of a database to share information between federal and state programs, and higher penalties and increased funding for fraud detection.

QUALITY INCENTIVES

- Patient-Centered Outcomes Research Institute was created to research different treatments and identify those that are most effective.
- Funding to states was increased for tort reform.
- A Medicare program was established to research bundled payments.
- An Independence at Home program was created to provide Medicare enrollees with home care with cost-sharing incentives for providers.
- A Medicare hospital value-based purchasing program was created to incentivize quality, which will also be expanded to home health companies and skilled nursing facilities.
- The Federal Coordinated Health Care Office was created within the Centers for Medicare and Medicaid Services to focus on dual eligible enrollees (those eligible for both Medicare and Medicaid) to improve care coordination between the states and the federal government. Health homes were established for Medicaid enrollees with chronic health issues to improve care.
- Medicaid fee-for-service payments for primary care providers were increased to Medicare rates for 2013 and 2014.
- Medicare provided a 10% bonus to primary care providers from 2011 to 2015.
- A national quality improvement strategy was created to choose quality measures, improve population health, improve the delivery of care, and improve patient outcomes.

- The Community-based Collaborative Care Network Program was created to improve care coordination for low-income uninsured and underinsured.
- Financial relationships must be disclosed between hospitals, physicians, other health care providers, pharmacists, and pharmacologic and medical device companies.

Preventive Services

- The National Prevention, Health Promotion and Public Health Council was created to coordinate public health initiatives at the federal level.
- The Prevention and Public Health Fund was created to finance these initiatives, conduct research, health screenings, and immunizations.
- Task forces were created for Preventive Services and Community Preventive Services to distribute information on preventive services.
- A grant program was created to promote wellness and prevention services targeting rural areas. The cost sharing for preventive services covered under Medicare was removed.
- An annual health risk assessment is covered under Medicare.

Long-term Care Programs

- The Community Living Assistance Services and Supports program was a voluntary insurance program to help individuals remain in the community instead of in a nursing home or other residence. It was repealed by the American Taxpayer Relief Act of 2012. The states are able to provide Medicaid coverage to those receiving home and community-based services through a state plan.
- The Community First Choice Option allows Medicaid to provide community-based services to those with disabilities who would otherwise be institutionalized. Skilled nursing facilities are required to disclose standardized information to Medicare to allow comparison between facilities.

COURT CHALLENGES

The ACA has withstood multiple court challenges to many different areas of the law. What follows explains the most important cases until the date of this publication.

Thomas More Law Center, et al, v. Barack H. Obama, President of the United States, et al

This case was decided on June 29, 2011, by the United States Court of Appeals for the Sixth Circuit. The Plaintiffs argued that the individual mandate was unconstitutional and that the ACA violated the right to free religion under the First

Amendment. The United States Court of Appeals for the Sixth Circuit ruled that the individual mandate was constitutional.

Virginia, ex rel. Kenneth T. Cuccinelli, II, Attorney General of Virginia v. Kathleen Sebelius, Secretary of Health and Human Services; Liberty University, et al, v. Timothy F. Geithner, Secretary of the Treasury, et al

These cases were decided on September 8, 2011, by the United States Court of Appeals for the Fourth Circuit. The Plaintiffs for the first case argued that the individual mandate was unconstitutional. The Plaintiffs for the second case argued that the ACA violated the First Amendment, they opposed federally funded abortions under the ACA, and they claimed that the ACA violated the guarantee of a Republican form of government under the Constitution. These cases were dismissed by the United States Court of Appeals for the Fourth Circuit on procedural grounds.

National Federation of Independent Business, et al, v. Kathleen Sebelius, Secretary of Health and Human Services, et al; Department of Health and Human Services, et al, v. Florida, et al; Florida, et al, v. Department of Health and Human Services, et al

These cases were decided on June 28, 2012, by the US Supreme Court. The Plaintiffs included the National Federation of Independent Businesses and 26 states who argued that the individual mandate and the Medicaid expansion were unconstitutional. The Supreme Court ruled that the individual mandate was constitutional. It ruled that it was unconstitutional to require states to participate in the Medicaid expansion or lose all of their federal funding for Medicaid. Therefore, this left it up to the states to decide whether they wished to participate in the Medicaid expansion.

Burwell v. Hobby Lobby Stores, Inc

This case was formally called *Hobby Lobby Stores, Inc. v. Sebelius*. It was decided on June 30, 2014, by the US Supreme Court. The Plaintiff argued against the contraceptive mandate in the ACA, which requires employers to provide coverage for contraception. The Supreme Court ruled that for-profit companies are exempt from a regulation if it violates the owner's religious beliefs, as long as there is a less restrictive way to further the interest of the law. Thus, the court ruled in favor of Hobby Lobby and struck down the contraceptive mandate.

Zubik v. Burwell; Priests for Life v. Burwell; Southern Nazarene University v. Burwell; Geneva College v. Burwell; Roman Catholic Archbishop of Washington v. Burwell; East Texas Baptist University v. Burwell; Little Sisters of the Poor Home for the Aged v. Burwell

These seven cases were consolidated and then decided on May 16, 2016, by the US Supreme Court. The Plaintiffs argued against the contraceptive mandate under the ACA. The Supreme Court ruled that the cases would return to the lower courts for reconsideration. On October 6, 2017, the Trump Administration issued rules that the contraception mandate did not have to be followed for religious or moral reasons. On October 16, 2017, the Plaintiffs settled with the Department of Justice, which allowed religious organizations not to provide coverage for items they were morally against.

FUTURE OF THE AFFORDABLE CARE ACT

With the election of President Trump, the future of the ACA under the current administration is uncertain. As of this publication, Republicans have been unsuccessful in their attempts to repeal and/or replace the ACA in its entirety. However, the Trump Administration has been able to make many changes to the ACA. Some important changes are noted here:

- January 11, 2018: States can impose work requirements for able-bodied Medicaid enrollees
- December 22, 2017: The Tax Cuts and Jobs Act repealed the individual mandate, which will go into effect in 2019
- October 12, 2017: Executive order signed allowing association health plans (plans offered by entities such as small businesses and trade associations) to be purchased across state lines, be formed by more groups, and require coverage for preexisting conditions; and ended the cost-sharing reduction subsidy payments to insurers who lowered copayments and deductibles for low-income enrollees, thus ensuring higher out-of-pocket costs for low-income patients
- October 6, 2017: Rules issued stating the contraception mandate did not have to be followed for religious or moral reasons

The only thing certain about Obamacare's future is uncertainty. Changing government regulations will have a wide-reaching effect throughout the health care industry. We (the authors) will not attempt to make any predictions regarding the ACA's future. Our goal is to provide you (the reader) with the facts regarding the background of this landmark piece of legislation.

Recommended Resources

Amadeo K. Donald Trump on health care: how Trump's health care policies will raise premium prices for you. The Balance. https://www.thebalance.com/how-could-trump-change-health-care-in-america-4111422. Updated April 16, 2018. Accessed April 20, 2018.

American Health Lawyers Association. Challenges to ACA at the U.S. Supreme Court. https://www.healthlawyers.org/Members/PracticeGroups/TaskForces/HRE/Pages/I._Challenges_to_ACA_at_the_US_Supreme_Court.aspx. Accessed April 20, 2018.

Ballotpedia. *Zubik v. Burwell.* https://ballotpedia.org/Zubik_v._Burwell#Decision. Accessed April 20, 2018.

Capretta JC, Antos JR. Indexing in the Affordable Care Act: the impact on the federal budget. Mercatus Research. https://www.mercatus.org/system/files/Capretta-Indexing-ACA.pdf. Published October 2015. Accessed April 20, 2018.

Centers for Medicare and Medicaid Services. Information on essential health benefits (EHB) benchmark plans. CMS.gov. https://www.cms.gov/cciio/resources/data-resources/ehb.html. Accessed April 20, 2018.

Centers for Medicare and Medicaid Services. Medical loss ratio. CMS.gov. https://www.cms.gov/CCIIO/Programs-and-Initiatives/Health-Insurance-Market-Reforms/Medical-Loss-Ratio.html. Accessed April 20, 2018.

Centers for Medicare and Medicaid Services. Reinsurance, risk corridors, and risk adjustment final rule. CMS.gov. https://www.cms.gov/CCIIO/Resources/Files/Downloads/3rs-final-rule.pdf. Published March, 2012. Accessed April 20, 2018.

Health Care Lawsuits. *Liberty University, Inc. et al v. Geithner et al.* http://www.healthcarelawsuits.org/detail.php?c=2276166&t=Liberty-University%2C-Inc.-et-al-v.-Geithner-et-al. Accessed April 20, 2018.

Health Care Lawsuits. *Thomas More Law Center v. President of the United States.* http://www.healthcarelawsuits.org/detail.php?c=2276356&t=Thomas-More-Law-Center-v.-President-of-the-United-States. Accessed April 20, 2018.

Hobby Lobby. The decision. http://hobbylobbycase.com/the-case/the-decision/. Accessed April 20, 2018.

Kaiser Family Foundation. How do Medicaid disproportionate share hospital (DSH) payments change under the ACA? https://kaiserfamilyfoundation.files.wordpress.com/2013/11/8513-how-do-medicaid-dsh-payments-change-under-the-aca.pdf. Published November 2013. Accessed April 20, 2018.

Kaiser Family Foundation. Status of state action on the Medicaid expansion decision. https://www.kff.org/health-reform/state-indicator/state-activity-around-expanding-medicaid-under-the-affordable-care-act/?activeTab=map&currentTimeframe=0&selectedDistributions=current-status-of-medicaid-expansion-decision&sortModel=%7B%22colId%22:%22Location%22,%22sort%22:%22asc%22%7D. Accessed April 20, 2018.

Kaiser Family Foundation. Summary of the Affordable Care Act. http://www.kff.org/health-reform/fact-sheet/summary-of-the-affordable-care-act/. Published April 25, 2013. Accessed April 20, 2018.

Leaming J. Virginia AG's lawsuit to scuttle landmark health care law dealt setback. American Constitution Society. https://www.acslaw.org/acsblog/all/commonwealth-of-virginia-v.-sebelius. Published September 8, 2011. Accessed April 20, 2018.

Mach AL. Excise tax on high-cost employer-sponsored health coverage: in brief. Congressional Research Service. https://fas.org/sgp/crs/misc/R44147.pdf. Published March 24, 2016. Accessed April 20, 2018.

Sheen R. ACA health insurance marketplace may stabilize in 2018. *The ACA Times*. https://acatimes.com/aca-health-insurance-marketplace-may-stabilize-in-2018/. Published January 22, 2018. Accessed April 20, 2018.

Supreme Court of the United States Blog. *Zubik v. Burwell*. http://www.scotusblog.com/case-files/cases/zubik-v-burwell/. Accessed April 20, 2018.

Supreme Court of the United States. Patient protection and Affordable Care Act cases. https://www.supremecourt.gov/docket/PPAACA.aspx. Accessed April 20, 2018.

Swendiman KS. Selected issues related to the effect of NFIB v. Sebelius on the Medicaid expansion requirements in section 2001 of the Affordable Care Act. Congressional Research Service. http://www.ncsl.org/documents/health/aca_medicaid_expansion_memo_1.pdf. Published July 16, 2012. Accessed April 20, 2018.

Uberoi N, Finegold K, Gee E. Health insurance coverage and the Affordable Care Act, 2010-2016. Department of Health and Human Services, Office of the Assistant Secretary for Planning and Evaluation. https://aspe.hhs.gov/system/files/pdf/187551/ACA2010-2016.pdf. Published March 3, 2016. Accessed April 20, 2018.

17

Spotting the Horizon
Future Directions in Health Care

Christopher A. Clyne, MD, MBA
Britton Jewell, DO, MHA

We hope that this book has provided you with a broad overview of the business of medicine. We believe that understanding these basic business concepts will make you an informed practitioner and will allow you to use this information to better care for your patients.

Even with this background knowledge, the only thing certain about the future of health care in the United States is uncertainty. However, we believe that there are some basic principles and trends that will continue in the future and withstand the test of time and political change. This chapter does not provide any guarantees or endorsements about the future of medicine or for any political party or affiliation.

There are several trends in the health care industry that are likely to continue to grow:

- Value-Based Care: Higher quality at a lower cost
- Risk-Based Arrangements: Reimbursement based on outcomes instead of episodic care or fee-for-service, such as accountable care organizations and increased use of bundled payments
- Utilization of Home- and Community-Based Services: More care provided outside of hospital settings and delay in institutionalization of patients in long-term care settings
- Advanced Practitioners: Increased need for advanced nursing practitioners and physician assistants, especially in primary care settings

- Big Data: The collection, pooling, sharing, and analyzing of large volumes of health information to improve population health
- Technology: Improvement and increased utilization of electronic health records, telemedicine, and home monitoring systems
- Large Health Systems: Vertical and horizontal growth of large health systems to include hospitals, insurers, skilled nursing facilities, home health agencies, physician groups, pharmacies, labs, researchers, and so on
- Hospitalists: Increased need and utilization of hospital-based physicians to provide expert care for hospitalized patients

This list is by no means all inclusive; however, it does provide some general ideas of where health care is currently going and will likely continue to move. With our ever-changing political environment, the future of the Affordable Care Act remains in question. The Trump Administration's repeal of the individual mandate has yet to go into effect. It is likely that the Medicaid expansion will remain despite attempts at repeal. It is unlikely that the current political climate and insurance industry would favor a single-payer system.

In conclusion, our health care system will continue to change, grow, and evolve, but will never stray from the ultimate goal of providing the best care for every individual. We hope that this book has expanded your knowledge and will serve as a useful resource for you in delivering high-quality patient care as you wrestle with the entanglements and requirements of the business of medicine.

Directory of State Board Websites

Alabama

Alabama Board of Medical Examiners
www.albme.org

Alaska

Alaska State Medical Board
www.commerce.alaska.gov/web/cbpl/ProfessionalLicensing/State
MedicalBoars.aspx

Arizona

Arizona Board of Osteopathic Examiners in Medicine and Surgery
www.azdo.gov

Arizona Medical Board
www.azmd.gov

Arkansas

Arkansas State Medical Board
www.armedicalboard.org

California

Medical Board of California
www.mbc.ca.gov

Osteopathic Medical Board of California
www.ombc.ca.gov

Colorado

Colorado Medical Board
www.colorado.gov/pacific/dora/Medical_Board

Connecticut

Connecticut Department of Public Health
https://portal.ct.gov/dph

Delaware

Delaware Board of Medical Licensure and Discipline
www.dpr.delaware.gov

District of Columbia

District of Columbia Board of Medicine
doh.dc.gov/bomed

Florida

Florida Board of Medicine
flboardofmedicine.gov

Florida Board of Osteopathic Medicine
floridasosteopathicmedicine.gov

Georgia

Georgia Composite Medical Board
medicalboard.georgia.gov

Hawaii

Hawaii Medical Board
cca.hawaii.gov/pvl

Idaho

Idaho Board of Medicine
bom.idaho.gov

Illinois

Illinois Department of Financial and Professional Regulation
https://www.idfpr.com/

Indiana

Medical Licensing Board of Indiana
www.in.gov/pla/medical.htm

Iowa

Iowa Board of Medicine
www.medicalboard.iowa.gov

Kansas

Kansas State Board of Healing Arts
www.ksbha.org

Kentucky

Kentucky Board of Medical Licensure
kbml.ky.gov

Louisiana

Louisiana State Board of Medical Examiners
www.lsbme.la.gov

Maine

Maine Board of Licensure in Medicine
www.maine.gov/md

Maine Board of Osteopathic Licensure
www.maine.gov/osteo

Maryland

Maryland Board of Physicians
www.mbp.state.md.us

Massachusetts

Massachusetts Board of Registration in Medicine
www.mass.gov/massmedboard

Michigan

Michigan Board of Medicine
www.michigan.gov/healthlicense

Michigan Board of Osteopathic Medicine and Surgery
www.michigan.gov/healthlicense

Minnesota

Minnesota Board of Medical Practice
mn.gov/boards/medical-practice

Mississippi

Mississippi State Board of Medical Licensure
www.msbml.ms.gov

Missouri

Missouri Board of Registration for the Healing Arts
pr.mo.gov/healingarts.asp

Montana

Montana Board of Medical Examiners
www.medicalboard.mt.gov

Nebraska

Nebraska Board of Medicine and Surgery
http://dhhs.ne.gov/publichealth/Pages/crl_crlindex.aspx

Nevada

Nevada State Board of Medical Examiners
medboard.nv.gov

Nevada State Board of Osteopathic Medicine
www.osteo.state.nv.us

New Hampshire

New Hampshire Board of Medicine
https://www.oplc.nh.gov/index.htm

New Jersey

New Jersey State Board of Medical Examiners
www.njconsumeraffairs.gov

New Mexico

New Mexico Board of Osteopathic Medical Examiners
www.rld.state.nm.us/boards/Osteopathy.aspx

New Mexico Medical Board
www.nmmb.state.nm.us

New York

New York State Board for Medicine
www.op.nysed.gov

North Carolina

North Carolina Medical Board
www.ncmedboard.org

North Dakota

North Dakota Board of Medicine
www.ndbom.org

Ohio

State Medical Board of Ohio
http://www.med.ohio.gov/

Oklahoma

Oklahoma Board of Medical Licensure and Supervision
www.okmedicalboard.org

Oklahoma State Board of Osteopathic Examiners
www.ok.gov/osboe

Oregon

Oregon Medical Board
www.oregon.gov/omb

Pennsylvania

Pennsylvania State Board of Medicine
www.dos.pa.gov/ProfessionalLicensing/BoardsCommissions/
Medicine/Pages/default.aspx

Pennsylvania State Board of Osteopathic Medicine
www.dos.pa.gov/ProfessionalLicensing/BoardsCommissions/
OsteopathicMedicine/Pages/default.aspx

Rhode Island

Rhode Island Board of Medical Licensure and Discipline
www.health.ri.gov

South Carolina

South Carolina Board of Medical Examiners
www.llr.state.sc.us/pol/medical

South Dakota

South Dakota Board of Medical and Osteopathic Examiners
www.sdbmoe.gov

Tennessee

Tennessee Board of Medical Examiners
https://www.tn.gov/health/health-program-areas/health-professional-boards/
me-board.html

Tennessee Board of Osteopathic Examination
https://www.tn.gov/health/health-program-areas/health-professional-boards/
osteo-board.html

Texas
Texas Medical Board
www.tmb.state.tx.us

Utah
Utah Division of Occupational and Professional Licensing
www.dopl.utah.gov

Vermont
Vermont Board of Medical Practice
healthvermont.gov/hc/med_board/bmp.aspx

Vermont Board of Osteopathic Physicians and Surgeons
www.sec.state.vt.us/professional-regulation/list-of-professions/
osteopathic-physicians.aspx

Virginia
Virginia Board of Medicine
www.dhp.virginia.gov

Washington
Washington Board of Osteopathic Medicine and Surgery
www.doh.wa.gov/LicensesPermitsandCertificates/ProfessionsNew
ReneworUpdate/OsteopathicPhysician

Washington Medical Quality Assurance Commission
www.doh.wa.gov

West Virginia
West Virginia Board of Medicine
https://wvbom.wv.gov/

West Virginia Board of Osteopathic Medicine
https://www.wvbdosteo.org/

Wisconsin
Wisconsin Medical Examining Board
https://dsps.wi.gov/Pages/Professions/Physician/Default.aspx

Wyoming
Wyoming Board of Medicine
wyomedboard.wyo.gov

Directory of States Requiring Controlled Substance License

Alabama

Connecticut

Delaware

District of Columbia

Hawaii

Idaho

Illinois

Indiana

Iowa

Louisiana

Maryland

Massachusetts

Michigan

Missouri

Nevada

New Jersey

New Mexico

Oklahoma

Rhode Island

South Carolina

South Dakota

Utah

Wyoming

Index